THE MEANING OF BDSM EXPERIENCES

The Meaning of BDSM Experiences

A Psychodynamic Perspective

Kandice van Beerschoten

<teneo> //press

AMHERST, NEW YORK

ISBN: 978-1-934844-54-0

TABLE OF CONTENTS

ACKNOWLEDGEMENTS

I am grateful to many people who provided support, guidance, and wisdom along this journey. First, a special thank you to those who participated in this study and opened up both their lives and homes to me. To those in the BDSM community, both friends and strangers, who opened doors so that I could recruit participants, your help is greatly appreciated. Jennifer Tolleson expertly guided me through the often difficult process of navigating a large volume of data and helped me gain clarity when all was muddled. R. Dennis Shelby understood the finer points and never failed to challenge me in new and unique ways. Sue Cebulko provided excellent advice and calmed me during the interview process when I faced an unexpected challenge. Lynne Tylke, whose early challenge to me to deepen my clinical thinking, had a profound influence on my ability to analyze and interpret the data. Denise Tsioles stepped in at the last minute and gave valuable feedback. All of you have guided me at various points along the way, and your words of wisdom have remained with me far beyond this project.

To my family: Alex and Krista, you have both been so patient and understanding to be so young. You both continue to teach me new things every day, and I am incredibly thankful for you. Most importantly, to my husband Stephan, thank you for your love, encouragement, and support. I am very fortunate to be your wife.

Finally, thank you to the many friends who have provided encouragement and support throughout this process. I am such a blessed person to have all of you in my life.

-KvB

THE MEANING OF BDSM EXPERIENCES

CHAPTER 1

INTRODUCTION

FORMULATION OF THE PROBLEM

This study explored what it means to be a heterosexual man living in the rural South who identifies as a "Dominant" within the BDSM community. BDSM (Bondage and discipline/Dominance and submission/sadism and masochism) has been a recognized, though curiously regarded, aspect of sexuality for centuries. In the United States, it continues to be seen as "kinky." The South, particularly rural areas trending more toward conservative values and mores, has a noted history of being weak in sexual research and strong in religious beliefs regarding sexual relations. Additionally, the activities that occur within BDSM have been labeled by the psychoanalytic community as "perverse."

The prevalence of BDSM within the United States is difficult to gauge, as this is an activity in which people may be reluctant to acknowledge participation. Estimates are that somewhere between 5 – 10% of the population participate in at least occasional sexual sadomasochism (Lowe, 1983) and 11 – 14% have experimented with BDSM at some point in their lives (Kleinplatz & Moser, 2007).

This study looked at two areas that would benefit from additional research: BDSM and southern sexuality. As Wilson (2006) states:

> Little concrete social science evidence exists . . . for evaluating the uniqueness of sexual attitudes and behaviors among Southerners, despite widespread attention to the study of human sexuality in the 20th century. Many social science researchers either do not control for or do not consider regional differences in analyzing their data (p. 164, "Sexuality").

Therefore, I hoped that selecting a sample from the rural South could bring a regional and cultural perspective that may prove valuable to sexuality studies.

While there is a great deal of psychoanalytic literature on sado-masochism, there is little research on what BDSM means subjectively to those who participate. Without this, there is a gap between what has been learned from research, theory, and practice. It was my hope that learning more about the internal world of this population would provide needed insight and contribute to the discussion regarding psychopathology. Additionally, the ideas and beliefs that clinicians hold about perversions and the people that are felt to be perverse are challenged as these categories become more clearly defined. Clinicians' understanding could be significantly deepened regarding the ways in which this community think about and experience their sexuality. By discovering the meanings that participants in BDSM assign to their sexual practices, the therapeutic experiences of BDSM participants may be positively affected.

BACKGROUND ON THE SOUTH

The history of the South is filled with suffering, most notably slavery, segregation, and war. However, there are positive aspects as well, including the stereotypically polite yet friendly quality that remains a part of Southern society today (Wilson, 2006). God, family and food seem to be a way of life for many, with Norman (2007) observing about the South that "the two-way flow between church and family is often expressed in food" (p. 97). Gender-driven manners and mannerisms also continue to be an integral part of Southern culture, with one expectation being that men and women will behave as "gentlemen" and "ladies." Throughout the South, children have been taught to answer with "sir" or "ma'am" (Olsen, 2009). When these various expectations are not met, it reflects poorly on that person's character. These manners signify dignity, respect for oneself and others, and adherence to an unspoken moral code that accompanies the external behaviors (Wilson, 2006).

Religion is another aspect of Southern life that holds a great deal of importance. In the South, the predominant religion is Christianity, with the overwhelming majority of Southerners identifying as Baptist (Kosmin & Mayer, 2001). In their articles of faith, the Southern Baptist Convention supports the books of Ephesians ("Wives, submit yourselves unto your own husbands, as unto the Lord;" chapter 5, verse 22) and Colossians ("Wives, submit yourselves unto your own husbands, as it is fit unto the Lord;" chapter 3, verse 18). In their family statement, the Southern Baptist Convention declares:

> The husband and wife are of equal worth before God, since both are created in God's image. The marriage relationship models the way God relates to His people. A husband is to love his wife as Christ loved the church. He has the God-given responsibility to provide for, to protect, and to lead his family. A wife is to submit herself graciously to the servant leadership of her husband even as the church willingly submits to the headship of Christ. She, being in the image of God as is her husband and thus equal to him, has the God-given responsibility to respect her husband and to serve as his helper in managing the household and nurturing the next generation ("The Family," para. 3).

Though a statement of equality is initially made, it is immediately negated by placing the husband in a dominant position above the wife. Also, due to the religious connotations involved, people may feel unable to behave or uncomfortable behaving in a contradictory manner because, as Hill (2006) notes, to disobey what is taught to be an "all-loving, all-requiring God," may bring feelings of shame or fear that one will go to Hell (p. 13, "Seriousness of Southern Religion"). The Bible tells men to be dominant and women to be submissive; therefore, this edict must be followed. These religious attitudes are particularly relevant to the rural South, as small country churches are where Southern evangelical churches first began (Flynt, 2006) .

This religious framework for how men and women should interact with each other brings forth gender roles embedded in paternalism. There is an air of inequality, lesser class and false protection (Olsen, 2009). There is no guarantee of respect or affection for the person in the "lower" position with this model. While boys are taught to be fiercely protective of their mothers (Olsen, 2009), they may still see their fathers being forcefully dominant in the home.

BACKGROUND ON BDSM

This culture of domination and submission based on religious attitudes interestingly resembles the BDSM community. This is a complex culture and difficult for those uninvolved to understand the intricacies. These practices have been part of societies for many centuries. Perhaps the first famous practitioner of BDSM was the Marquis de Sade, the figure for which "sadism" was named (Blanchot, 1965; Warren, 2000). He wrote fictional stories depicting torturous tales of sexual bondage and beatings, often by fictitious religious or political figures, prompting Napoleon Bonaparte to order his arrest. Literary critics over time have determined his work to be more philosophical than perverse (Moore, 1995).

Within the BDSM subculture of Dominance and submission (or D/s), there is a voluntary, consensual surrender of power by a submissive to a Dominant. Dominants do not take power from an unwilling partner but rather wait for this to be given to them. Warren (2000) calls consent "a touchstone, an axiom, a sacrament" (p. 33), stating, "it must be constantly present and mutually respected within the relationship" (p. 33).

Two key dynamics within D/s relationships are that of power and control. Though many D/s relationships do usually include aspects of sadomasochism, it is often referred to as the 'mental side' of BDSM. Once a submissive gives control to a Dominant, a "power exchange" is said to occur, which typically lasts for the duration of the scene. These people are sometimes referred to as "players," while those who engage in a continuous power exchange are referred to as "24/7." Stoller (1991) also identified trust as an essential component, stating, "By far the most important element to be established is trust: these sadomasochists all appreciate sophisticated partners who know exactly how to play within the rules of the game while seeming – with exquisite nuance – to be exceeding the limits" (p. 19).

The idea of voluntary pain is difficult for some outside of BDSM to comprehend. While not all D/s relationships involve physical pain, many do incorporate it (Warren, 2000). The pain involved during a scene is not only consensual but is also negotiated prior to the scene to ensure the submissive's limits are known and respected. Smirnoff (1969) refers to the sadist in the relationship as "merely a slave of the self-styled victim" (para. 9) and then reminds the reader "we must not forget that it is the victim who lays down the rules" (para. 9). Weinberg (1995) adds that scenes are often planned in advance between partners, resulting in shared control. He also points out that, for some, pain is merely a method by which control is established. Moreover, the pain inflicted may not be experienced as suffering. Stoller (1991) describes how pain inflicted in one place on the body might feel pleasurable, yet if applied to a slightly different location, the feeling could be excruciating. Not all pain is erotic, even for a masochist.

Most modern practitioners of BDSM follow the edict of "Safe, Sane, and Consensual" (SSC), a term first introduced by David Stein (Downing, 2007). This means that that nothing will be done to endanger the health or well-being of another person, either physically or emotionally. To ensure this happens, a "safeword" is normally available for the submissive's use, signaling that the activity taking place has surpassed her limits and is no longer consensual. Once in a scene, Dominants follow cues from their submissives regarding her level of physical, psychological and sexual comfort. Warren (2000) notes that "the change in tone and body language as the submissive searches for the safeword is usually enough to warn a sensitive dominant that something is wrong" (p. 33). "Sane" warns against going outside the limits of the cultural norms by doing things that would be considered questionable or dangerous (Warren, 2000). Most importantly, both parties must consent not only to the relationship but to each individual act, much like normative sexuality.

An alternative to SSC is RACK or "Risk Aware Consensual Kink." The addition of this term allowed the BDSM community to move away from the potential implied psychopathology it had subjected itself to by inclusion of the term "sane" in SSC (Downing, 2007; Williams, Thomas, Prior, and Christiansen, 2014). It also allowed for community discourse on edgier forms of play about which no consensus could be reached about safety, such as sexual asphyxia (Downing, 2007). RACK advocates for informed consent of the activities that will take place, so that all parties are apprised of potential risks. It does indeed allow for more intense or edgier forms of play to occur within community norms.

A new proposed standard for BDSM play is known as the 4Cs: caring, communication, consent, and caution (Williams et al., 2014). Williams et al. (2014) state that consent "has often been thought of as a key element that distinguishes BDSM from violence and other types of abuse" (para. 1), and they distinguish between surface, scene, and deep consent. Communication is described an essential element within both relationships and scenes, as well as a "bridge between caring and caution" (para. 3). Caring invokes an "ethic of care" to help create an atmosphere of "safety, trust, and respect for our partners" (para.1). Caution "implies a need to be aware of risk, the possibility of danger, and an admonition to proceed carefully" (para 2).

Throughout this book, the term "perversion" will be used, and it is important to distinguish what is meant by this. Steiner (1982) used the word "perversion" to reference the perverse nature of relationships with others, as well as perverse aspects within parts of the self. Though he did note that these uses of the concept of perversion were likely linked to sexual perversions, sadomasochism in particular, his focus was more on relational and internal uses of the word rather than behavior that manifested as sexual (Steiner, 1982). McDougall (1986) also differentiates between these types of perversion, stating "it seems to me that the only aspect of a fantasy that might legitimately be described as perverse would be the attempt to force one's erotic fantasies on a non-consenting or a non-responsible other. Perhaps in the last resort only relationships may aptly be termed perverse" (p. 20). Therefore, this study confines the definition of "perversion" to behavior.

When the word "perversion" is used, it will be to reference sexual perversions and a mostly contemporary perspective will be employed with regard to this definition. In the psychoanalytic community, the word "perversion" has traditionally held a negative connotation. However, in more recent literature, aided by postmodernism, the ideas of scholars have begun to take a different form. Stoller (1991), who studied sadomasochists extensively, expressed his view of "perversion":

> Though studying the meaning of perversion is worthwhile, what counts far more is the basic question: How much harm does any individual, not just the sadomasochist, inflict on other living creatures: Actually inflict. Not just in imagination or in the theater of erotic behavior (as, for instance, that of the consensual sadomasochists). . . . Theater takes place on a stage, a construction in the real world or in our minds; and in that staging are placed safety factors allowing people to play out fantasies of harm, humilia-

tion, revenge, and triumph without actual harming, humiliating, revenging, or triumphing over others (pp. 48-49).

Dimen (2001) states that "perversion may be defined . . . as the sex that you like and I don't" (p. 827). She further elaborates:

> Homosexuality, for example, came off the diagnostic books a long time ago, even if in the minds of some people, including analysts, it remains a perversion. Maybe, as the stigma lifts from one marginal sexual practice, it doesn't disappear but alights on another— from homosexuality to b&d, from b&d to bloodletting, from bloodletting to—do visions of slippery slopes enter your minds (p. 827)?

Symington (2002), who likewise uses the example of homosexuality as previously stigmatized in the psychoanalytic community as perverse, also contributes his ideas about the definition of and what constitutes a perversion:

> The question of what is perverse and what is not can, I believe, only be solved by scrutinizing the emotional activity of which the sexual activity is a sign. Normality and perversity in sexual mores cannot be determined by the outer activity alone. Sexual intercourse between a man and a woman cannot be called normal just on the basis of the physical sexual act. If it is done with emotional tenderness, it is different from when it is done out of hostile vengeance. When we look at it in this way, the very words "normal" and "perverse" seem to come out of the wrong mindset (pp. 128-129).

Here, the focus shifts from the action alone to the emotional intent behind the behavior and the quality of the relationship. This study sought to discover precisely what those emotions and intentions were, as described by the participants, as well as the way the participant experienced emotional interactions with his partner, and then interpretively uncover the meaning of that. More specifically, the researcher sought to determine if the behaviors presented as pathological within these individuals.

PERSONAL PERSPECTIVES AND BIASES

I came to this study with two important and relevant personal biases. First, the research centered on a central concept of perversion, a topic of debate within the psychoanalytic community. Though some may view BDSM participation as perverse, I disagree with this. Indeed, I am a member of the BDSM community. This was a fact that I disclosed upfront to participants and understood as relevant to the lens through which I would be interpreting the data.

Second, I am a Caucasian woman who was born, raised, and has lived most of my life in the rural South. Having spent much of my career in a part of the South that is definitively rural (population 5800), I have seen how people live and the hardships they endure simply by virtue of the lack of access to resources (or even indoor plumbing). I have witnessed continuing racism and, as a woman, have been subjected to sexism and continuing paternalism. I did not have to specifically disclose to my participants that I was southern, as I feel certain my accent did this for me.

Even with her significant flaws, I cannot help my affection for the South. Given that all of my participants were men who were also raised in the South, I felt that this was an advantage. We shared two unique cultures: being southern and being members of the BDSM community. They could rest assured from the start that I would not judge them for either of these identifications. Both identifications gave me a certain amount of credibility. On multiple levels, I was "one of them."

Chapter 2

Literature Review

The heterosexual BDSM community challenges our ideas about and definitions of perversions. Are they indeed "perverse" or does a review of the literature lead to other conclusions? In an effort to elucidate our clinical assumptions about this community, literature was reviewed regarding sadism and masochism, reparation, identification, countertransference with BDSM-identified patients, and empirical studies.

PERVERSION

As pointed out by Dios Reis Filho et al. (2005), "The first difficulty is to define the concept of perversion: there is no unanimous point of view regarding this clinical manifestation among the different psychoanalytical schools." In the Dora case study, Freud (1905) noted perversion as "...instances in which the sexual function has extended its limits in respect either to the part of the body concerned or to the sexual object chosen" (p. 146). He elaborated on perversions in *Three Essays on the Theory of Sexuality* (1905) and separately discussed inversions and fetishes. However, he later refers to all three situations as being perverse. Further confusing readers was Freud's uncertainty when directly addressing the issue of whether or not homosexuality should be considered a perversion (1905).

Laplanche and Pontalis (1973) defined perversion in this way:

> Deviation from the "normal" sexual act when this is defined as coitus with a person of the opposite sex directed towards the achievement of orgasm by means of genital penetration. Perversion is said to be present; where the orgasm is reached with other sexual objects (homosexuality, pedophilia, bestiality, etc.) or through other regions of the body (anal coitus, etc.); where the orgasm is subordinated absolutely to certain extrinsic conditions, which may even be sufficient in themselves to bring about sexual pleasure (fetishism, transvestitism, voyeurism and exhibitionism, sado-masochism). In a more comprehensive sense, "perversion" connotes the whole of the psycho-sexual behaviour that accompanies such atypical means of obtaining sexual pleasure ("Perversion").

More recently, McDougall (2000) stated:

> The only sexual predilections that I would qualify as perverse are limited to certain forms of relationship to the other, notably sexual acts that do not take into account the needs or desires of the partner, such as sexual child abuse, rape, exhibitionism, and voyeurism, or necrophilia (frequently preceded by murder of the chosen partner) (The Question of "Perversion").

Dios Reis Filho et al. (2005) echoed this sentiment, stating, "We cannot describe as 'perversion' what two adults do privately, with mutual consent, to cheer up their sexual life. Also, it is not the fantasy that characterizes perversion; in other words, there is no difference between perverse and neurotic fantasies."

The terms "sadism" and "masochism" were first coined by Krafft-Ebing (1892), with sadism being derived from the French writer-philosopher Marquise de Sade, while masochism was taken from the name of the author von Sacher-Masoch, who tended toward the subject of masochism in his writing, as well as his personal life. In discussing sadism, while referring to it as a perversion, Krafft-Ebing also normalizes it by pointing out how normal sexual relations can spawn small acts of sadism, such as biting or wrestling. He explains this by stating that "lust and cruelty often occur together" and that this was not unusual (Krafft-Ebing, 1892). He explained the phenomenon of sadism:

> It is clear how lust impels to acts that otherwise are expressive of anger. The one, like the other, is a state of exaltation, an intense excitation of the whole psycho-motor sphere. Thus there arises an impulse to react on the object that induces the stimulus, in every possible way, and with the greatest intensity. Just as maniacal exaltation easily passes to furibund destructiveness, exaltation of the sexual emotion often induces an impulse to expend itself in senseless and apparently harmful acts. To a certain extent these are psychical accompaniments; but it is not simply an unconscious excitation of innervation of muscles (which also sometimes occurs as blind violence); it is a true hyperbulia, a desire to exert the most intense effect on the individual giving rise to the stimulus. The most intense means, however, is the infliction of pain (Krafft-Ebing, 1892, pp. 58-59).

Freud (1905) followed this up with his seminal *Three Essays on the Theory of Sexuality*, in which he called sadism and masochism "the most common and the most significant of all the perversions" (Sadism and Masochism). He defined sadism simply as "the desire to inflict pain upon the sexual object" (Sadism and Masochism), noting that the word alone brings with it the implication for the desire to subjugate and humiliate. When discussing the origins of sadism, Freud says:

> As regards . . . sadism, the roots are easy to detect in the normal. The sexuality of most male human beings contains an element of aggressiveness—a desire to subjugate; the biological significance of it seems to lie in the need for overcoming the resistance of the sexual object by means other than the process of wooing. Thus sadism would correspond to an aggressive component of the sexual instinct which has become independent and exaggerated

and, by displacement, has usurped the leading position (1905, Sadism and Masochism).

Masochism was defined as the "reverse" of sadism (Sadism and Masochism, para. 1), though he noted that masochism "seems to be further removed from the normal sexual aim than its counterpart" (Sadism and Masochism). Additionally, he agreed with Krafft-Ebing (1892) that sadism appears as the active form, while masochism takes the passive form (Freud, 1905).

While drawing no definitive conclusions on sadism and masochism in terms of pathology, Freud (1905) instead said that these capabilities are in everyone, though the extent to which they are developed varies "and may be increased by the influences of actual life" (p. 38). While not naming sadism and masochism specifically, there was the implication that he did not find these behaviors to be pathological in nature but on the normative side of sexuality (Freud, 1905).

While Freud initially theorized that sadism probably developed before masochism (Freud, 1905), he later reversed this, broaching the idea that, in the sadomasochism dyad, masochism is first formed and is primary (Freud, 1920b). Additionally, he states that sadism is a part of the death instinct that comes into the service of the libido. He asserts that a certain amount of aggression is necessary for the sexual act (Freud, 1920b).

In *A Child Is Being Beaten*, Freud (1920a) looked at adults who were having child beating fantasies and theorized about the possible etiology of sadistic fantasies. He stated that these fantasies seemed to appear in three phases. The first is represented by the phrase "My father is beating the child whom I hate," and this phase is sadistic in nature. With the second phase, the person reverts to masochism, unconsciously thinking "I am being beaten by my father," as the figures of the fantasies shift slightly. As guilt takes over, the third phase begins and restores sadism with the father being represented by another authority figure, and the adult observing once again as another child is beaten. Freud (1920a) is clear in his belief regarding the origins of both these fantasies and perversions:

> The perversion is no longer an isolated fact in the child's sexual life, but falls into its place among the typical, not to say normal, processes of development which are familiar to us. It is brought into relation with the child's incestuous object-love, with its Oedipus complex. It first comes into prominence in the sphere of this complex, and after the complex has broken down it remains over, often quite by itself, the inheritor of its store of libido, and weighed down by the sense of guilt that was attached to it. The abnormal sexual constitution, finally, has shown its strength by forcing the Oedipus complex into a particular direction, and by compelling it to leave an unusual residue behind.

He further added that the experience of pleasure during the masochistic oedipal fantasies is the cause of the resulting guilt. He concluded by stating that he hoped to "have raised an expectation that the sexual aberrations of childhood, as well as those of mature life, are ramifications of the [Oedipus] complex" (Freud, 1920a).

Several authors (Whitebook, 1991; Bak, 1974; Stoller, 1975; Roiphe and Galenson, 1987; and Gillespie, 1956) have noted the importance of castration anxiety in the consideration of perversions. If the developmental tasks of the Oedipal complex are not satisfactorily fulfilled, then this increases the possibility that the child will regress to the experience of castration anxiety (Gillespie, 1956). The emergence of perversions may then be a defensive response, with fetishes appearing to be the clearest example of this (Bak, 1974; Freud, 1927).

Clark (1927) approached this subject, taking note of others in the field who hypothesized that sadism originates in infancy during breastfeeding at the point during which the baby begins to teeth. During this time, the child will use mother's nipple as a teething aid, essentially, and derive pleasure from this, as well as from the pain that is inflicted upon her. However, Clark believes that sadism begins much earlier, particularly with the slight the infant feels at the trauma of physical separation due to birth. There is then another significant trauma, which occurs when the mother weans the child from the breast. He notes that the mother's decision to wean is a narcissistic one and that, in an effort to identify with the mother, the infant then adopts the mother's narcissistic attitude. The result is that the child gets to observe the mother's love being wounded by the child's behaviors, which is gratifying. This theory has the modern-day problem that many mothers now subscribe to the idea of child-led weaning, and there has been no report of a decrease in sadomasochistic activities.

More recently, Mollinger (1982) states that in the initial stage of development, the child holds a belief that if he sees himself as separate from the parent, then he will be annihilated. To prevent this from happening, the child identifies with the parent in order to maintain the relationship as closely as possible. This can result in sadism, masochism or both, depending on the parent's behavior. In a later stage, once the superego has developed, the child may feel guilty for oedipal desires and begin fantasizing about punishment as a way of coping, leading to the origin of sadomasochistic fantasies (Mollinger, 1982).

Stoller (1985), who did a great deal of ethnographic research in the sadomasochism community, stated a belief that any perverse act is an attempt to visit revenge upon traumas of the past. In what he terms "the script," the trauma ends differently for the victim, more successfully, so that the person no longer feels the emotional pain of the past. This is replaced with a sense of "triumph." For this reason, Stoller called sadomasochistic scenes "psychodramas," as he viewed them as reenactments of these psychological scripts (Stoller, 1985).

Several analysts view sadomasochism in terms of a continuum (Kernberg, 1991; Silverstein, 1994). Silverstein (1994) views sexuality with "mature object love with equality and reciprocity of power" at the healthy end of the spectrum and sadomasochism at the "unhealthy" opposite end. However, she offers no rationale for why these are mutually exclusive. She asserts that early object relations are the basis for later dominant sexual behavior, meaning dominant parental relationships may create sexual dominants. This makes up for the lack of power that is experienced as a toddler and essentially defends against the possible re-experiencing of submission. Kernberg (1998) held a similar line of thinking to Silverstein. He stated that various factors could potentially contribute to the formation of aggression, such as neurobiological imbalances, trauma (abuse, pain, illness) or unhealthy early object relationships. Early experiences with parents or caretakers that are felt as dominating/domineering, humiliating or sadistic may be factors in the child developing a perversion, such as sadism (Kernberg, 1998).

SADOMASOCHISM.

Freud (1905) addressed the reciprocity between emotional sadism and masochism, stating that "it can often be shown that masochism is nothing more than an extension of sadism turn round up on the subject's own self" (p. 26). He states that the unique aspect of sadism and masochism as perversions is that they always occur simultaneously in the same person. The question remains as to how well-developed each side is in each individual.

The dyadic nature of sadism and masochism, leading them to be blended into the singular word "sadomasochism," has been noted by others as well. Ellis (1995) notes that "sadism and masochism may be regarded as complementary emotional states; they cannot be regarded as opposed states" (p. 37).

In *Pain and Passion*, Stoller (1991) used interviews with members of the sexual sadomasochistic community to illustrate individual etiology, relational dynamics, and protocols. In particular, Stoller follows the relationship of Tammy and Dan. While Tammy is a professional Dominatrix by day, she submits to Dan, a Dominant, in their romantic relationship. However, Dan suffers a great deal emotionally during their tumultuous relationship, as he is placed in the masochist role due to her addiction and psychological issues. Stoller is able to illustrate through the interview transcripts that, while Tammy and Dan may have defined roles within their sexual dynamic where Dan is the one in control, this does not necessarily hold true for non-sexual aspects of their relationship. Dan is unable to control her drug addiction nor is he able to dominate her mind to the extent that she no longer has intrapsychic conflict. Their roles become reversed when not actively participating in the sexual aspects of BDSM (Stoller, 1991).

Silverstein (1994) also addressed the reciprocal roles of sadism and masochism, stating that "the ability to reverse roles in sexual fantasy is a form of empathy -- the capacity to experience what another experiences." However, she largely referred to fantasies instead of actual behavior.

FETISHISM DIFFERENTIATED FROM SEXUAL SADOMASOCHISM.

Freud (1905) addressed the issue of fetishes separately from that of sadism and masochism. He noted that the person with a fetish will at times have no desire for what is considered to be normal sex in favor of contact with the overvalued replacement sexual object. In cases of pathological behavior, the person is unable to achieve sexual satisfaction or arousal without the replacement object. In the case of sadomasochism, sexual aim, while normally still achieved, is delayed by the administration or reception of pain (Freud, 1905).

It is this main difference, aim versus object, which has continued to keep these two sexual variations clinically separate through the years. Both the DSM and the International Classification of Diseases (ICD) have them listed as individual disorders, with no features shared between them (Reiersol and Skeid, 2006).

However, the BDSM community is frequently associated synonymously with the fetish community (NLA-I Media Statement Regarding Consensual SM, 2008). While the two can intermingle, depending on individual preferences, this is not meant to indicate that all BDSM practitioners have a fetish or vice versa. Indeed, the word "fetish" has become a colloquial way for even those within the BDSM community to refer to activities

PERVERSIONS PATHOLOGIZED.

Though perversions began with the recognition that everyone has these impulses and this dark side to a certain extent (Freud, 1905), over time, perversions began to be seen through a more pathological lens.

It is difficult to say exactly when this was or if there was a specific event that facilitated this. However, Stoller (1985) notes that, in 1952, the original DSM, under Sexual Deviation, listed "and sexual sadism (including rape, sexual assault, mutilation)" (p. 5). Masochism was not listed. In 1968, when the DSM-II was released, the qualifier at the end was removed, giving wide berth for interpretations, both correct and incorrect. Additionally, masochism was added as a disorder at this time (Stoller, 1985). The addition of sadism and masochism as mental disorders would have logically furthered any beliefs that these behaviors were pathological in nature. However, given the works of various contributors to this discussion (Krafft-Ebing, 1892; Ellis, 1995; Freud, 1905, 1920b), it seems there is sufficient evidence that some believed sadism was pathological behavior years before the DSM was published.

More recently, Bollas (1984) also discusses the issue of how emotions interact with perversions. He writes about different types of relationships in which hate is the predominate way of interacting. However, the hate he refers to is not meant to destroy the object but rather to sustain it. He refers to this form of hate as "an unconscious form of love" (p. 2). The important thing for the person who hates is to get some sort of reaction from the object, even if that means retaliation. What would feel intolerable would be to be ignored. He stresses that loving hate can be "a defense against emptiness" (p. 9). With regard to loving hate as a form of perversion, he references Stoller's (1975) belief that the erotic form of hatred defines perversion. He also sides with Khan's belief that perversion includes a significant element of dehumanization, which ultimately (and in blanket fashion) pathologizes perversion. Bollas does not appear to believe that loving hate is a perversion. He believes that with perversions, there is a clear intention to harm the object, while the opposite is true of loving hate. He also states that people seek to avoid affective states through the enactment of perversions, while loving hate is giving in to those affective states. He is careful to separate loving hate from the perversions (Bollas, 1984).

Stoller (1985) sees perversions as the avoidance of intimacy. He elaborates that the desire to harm the erotic object choice is a form of dehumanization, as true intimacy is not possible given the psychological dynamics involved in vengeful acts (Stoller, 1985). However, Stoller (1991) explains well the idea behind sadomasochistic pain, which is experienced as pleasure, and how this differs greatly from ordinary pain, which is still felt as actual pain and is unpleasant, even for the masochist.

In *The Bonds of Love*, Benjamin (1988) uses *Story of O* as her basis for discerning how BDSM relationships function. Benjamin discounts the fact of consent throughout the book, taking the point of view that there is only objectivity and no subjectivity in BDSM relationships. She states that "domination...is a twisting of the bonds of love. For the person who takes this route to establishing his own power, there is an absence where the other should be" (p. 219). She further elaborates:

> Thus, beginning, with the first relationship – of parent and child – we note the uneasy coexistence of contradictory tendencies: mutual recognition and unequal complementarity. We observe how complementarity subsumes mutuality in erotic domination, where the idea of a powerful person acting on a powerless one inspires the thrill of a transgression (Benjamin, 1988, p. 222).

Even with the element of consent, however, this does not mean that all acts of sadism are normal. In what appears to be a clear description of pathological sadism, Jukes (1993) attempts to describe the mentality of men who abuse the female partners:

Men need to dominate in order to ensure that women are available as this object of fantasy—sexually in particular. When woman refuses to be controlled, either by asserting her independence or by frustrating men's expectations, the man is in danger of falling into the gap, the point of non-existence. This peril is associated with talion sadistic and homicidal rage directed at the historically constructed cause, the feminine. When he fails to control her, he becomes violent because he cannot tolerate seeing the emptiness on his other side. The phallus, which assumes its importance from its absence on a woman, is the symbol of domination, and the erect penis is its instrument. The Oedipus complex structures the erection as the instrument of male domination, and the only potential for intimacy through the eroticization of dominance in heterosexuality. Woman has—is—nothing.

This evidences the misogyny that is often thought to be involved in traditional gender BDSM relationships.

Richards (2003) pathologizes perversion by stating that she believes it to be "a source of pleasures that induce a person to devalue the pleasures of making love" (p. 2). She acknowledges that a certain amount of sadomasochistic behavior is present in all relationships. She outlines what she sees as several key elements of perversion:

1. Valuing a particular scenario, animal, inanimate object, or part of a person more than another person's happiness or approval;
2. compulsion;
3. sexual pleasure and pleasure in the discharge of aggression;
4. shame and attendant grandiosity; and
5. coercion masquerading as love (Richards, 2003, p. 2).

In the discussion on sadomasochism and pathology, several writers have noted the involvement of narcissism. Clark (1920) stated that the idea of treatment is to "break down the [narcissism] and place more libido to the service of love objects" (p. 3). More recently, others (Kernberg, 1991; Leonoff, 1997) have linked sadism to narcissistic characterology, as well.

Leonoff (1997) discussed the connection between sadism and narcissism from a vantage point of severe pathology. He aligned sadism, which he views as a defense, and what Kernberg (1991) would call malignant narcissism, stating that the two intermingle when the submission of the object to the sadist reinforces his omnipotence. Further, Leonoff (1997) asserted that the sadist experiences "triumph, not simply over the object but over the very idea of limits itself. In this regard, the sadist cathects death in order to become its master" (p. 4). He then goes on to discuss the link between sadism and murder, stating that, "there is an inherent risk in all sadistic perversion that murderous impulses may actually break through erotic containment" (p. 4). While he acknowledged that limits are set by sexual sadomasochistic participants, this seems to be noted for the purpose of strengthening his argument that limits are necessary in order to prevent murderous impulses within a scene. Leonoff goes on to talk about sadism, using the torturous and sexualized murder of a child as a hypothetical situation. He concludes by discussing his own version of the aforementioned continuum, stating that mild narcissism is on one end of the spectrum and murder in the interest of "self-definition" is on the other (Leonoff, 1997).

PERVERSIONS DEPATHOLOGIZED.

In Freud's (1905) discussion of perversion in his *Three Essays on the Theory of Sexuality*, he addressed the issue of pathology. In particular, he looked at which perversions meet the standard of true pathology and which ones fall closer to normal sexuality. He said:

> Everyday experience has shown that most of these extensions, or at any rate the less severe of them, are constituents which are rarely absent from the sexual life of healthy people, and are judged by them no differently from other intimate events. If circumstances favour such an occurrence, normal people too can substitute a perversion of this kind for the normal sexual aim for quite a time, or can find place for the one alongside the other. No healthy

person, it appears, can fail to make some addition that might be called perverse to the normal sexual aim; and the universality of this finding is in itself enough to show how inappropriate it is to use the word perversion as a term of reproach. If a perversion, instead of appearing merely *alongside* the normal sexual aim and object, and only when circumstances are unfavourable to *them* and favourable to *it*—if, instead of this, it ousts them completely and takes their place in *all* circumstances—if, in short, a perversion has the characteristics of exclusiveness and fixation—then we shall usually be justified in regarding it as a pathological symptom (Freud, 1905, The Perversions in General).

Here, he seemed to support pathologizing most perversions only in situations where the person has situated their sexuality entirely within the realm of the perversion. If it becomes the only means by which sexual gratification can be achieved, then pathology exists. However, Freud (1905) did not appear to believe this to be the case for the vast majority of people experiencing perversions.

Ellis (1995) addressed the assumption that sadism is a defense through which true emotional connection can be avoided, which is a major connecting factor among those who pathologize sexually sadomasochistic behavior. Ellis (1995) makes the important distinction that love is an essential element in both the infliction and reception of pain, not cruelty, in both sadism and masochism. Largely, there is an emotional connection within these relationships. He also notes that sadists, like other partners, continue to be concerned with the sexual satisfaction of the masochists involved (Ellis, 1995).

Hodges (1961) takes a different approach, stating that since sadism repressed will be experienced as masochism, a lack of cruelty is what should be considered pathological. He discusses the differences between moral and immoral sadism, stating that most people, in general, are morally sadistic by gaining pleasure from the punishment that wrong-doers receive. Hodges believed moral sadism, which he situated in the superego, to be much more convenient. He also stated that immoral sadism, such as "disparaging and ridiculing the virtuous," could be liberating (Hodges, 1961).

Though she appears to believe sadomasochism to be pathological in nature, Benjamin (1988) gives a helpful description of the attunement necessary for and present in BDSM relationships with the concept of mutual recognition:

> Receptivity and self-expression, the sense of losing the self in the other and the sense of being truly known for oneself all coalesce. In my view, the simultaneous desire for loss of self and for wholeness (or oneness) with the other, often described as the ultimate point of erotic union, is really a form of the desire for recognition. In getting pleasure *with* the other and taking pleasure *in* the other, we engage in mutual recognition (p. 126).

This also describes the emotional connection of which Ellis (1995) speaks.

Kernberg (1991) looks at the different ways in which sadomasochism can be utilized. Two of the determinants in whether or not people transform their fantasies into behaviors are the composition of the superego and the extent to which they utilize splitting. Also holding the view that sadomasochistic behavior lies on a continuum, Kernberg illustrates various forms of sadomasochism, ranging from pathological sadism to BDSM within the context of a stable marriage. Under extremely pathological circumstances . . . the malignant recruitment of love at the service of aggression" is perversion (p. 5). Kernberg acknowledges that Freud's (1920a) theory behind perversions, regarding oedipal issues, continues to hold true. He states, "Erotic desire . . . permits the expression of sadomasochism as an unconventional, asocial, private, secret, intimate reconstitution of triumph over the oedipal couple in the primal scene" (p. 11). Kernberg (1991) notes that there is trust involved in both causing pain to a partner and in the reception of this pain.

Kernberg (1992) also attempts to define sadism and domination in terms of aggression. He calls sadism a "less severe degree of hatred" (p. 24).

He states that this can be expressed as a sexualized desire to inflict pain or it can come in the forms of narcissistic or sadomasochistic personality styles. It is noted that the goal is not to destroy either the relationship or the object but rather to maintain the relationship in order to continue fulfilling the desires of the sadist. Kernberg categorizes dominance as "a still milder form of hatred . . . a search for power over [the object]" (p. 24). He says that sadomasochism may or may not be a part of these relationships but that the object has ultimate control, as the dominant force can only have as much control as the submissive object will allow.

Kernberg (1992) notes that there is an "implied reconfirmation of the subject's freedom and autonomy" (p. 24) with this type of "hatred." This reference to dominance and the emphasis on the subject's continued autonomy are of particular interest here and are important to the issue of depathologizing the behaviors of Dominants.

McDougall (1986) raised the question of when perversions should be "regarded as a simple variation or version of adult sexuality and when is it to be judged symptomatic" (p. 29). Expressing the belief that "only relationships may aptly be termed perverse" (p. 29), she proposed alternative terminology.

> The term neosexualities is chosen to emphasize the innovative and somewhat unreal character of deviant sexual acts and relationships. These area response to incoherent communications and unconscious problems on the part of parents. The concept of addictive sexuality or neoneeds is also introduced in reference to the compulsivity that invariably accompanies perverse sexuality (pp. 29-30).

Along the lines of questioning whether perversion should be considered a symptom, Chodorow (1992) explored the possibility of heterosexuality as a compromise formation, and also stated that all sexualities are, in essence, a compromise formation. This mitigates the focus on BDSM, as well as other sexualities previously considered perverse, as a symptom. Hoffman (2000) reinforced this idea by applying the idea of compromise formation to mainstream sexual orientations – heterosexuality, homosexuality, and bisexuality.

Parsons (2000) notes that "both Glasser and McDougal . . . characterised perversion in terms of the quality of the relationship to the object" (p. 8). He further states that Freud's original idea of a drive consisting of source, aim and object should be "rephrased, to say that a drive consists of source, aim and quality of relatedness to object" (p. 9). Symington (2002) echoed this with his focus on the "emotional activity" of a couple instead of merely their manifest sexual behavior (p. 128).

Saketopoulou (2014), utilizing LaPlanche's theory of infantile sexuality, explores the developmental relationship between pleasure and pain, as well as how perversions "[*aspire*] to the unraveling of the ego (p. 263)." She also discusses how the analyst's ability to tolerate curious exploration of perverse sexuality can lead to resolution of generational psychical residue carried by the patient.

> The potential for transformation lies in the fact that, when revisited by a developmentally more mature subject, such signifiers can become reconfigured on the level of the body, thus allowing new life to be breathed into them. Instead of remaining inside the subject as sediments of the parental other they can be taken more into our own possession. That which has been intergenerationally injected into us can become assembled anew as it becomes rethreaded with personal bits of experience. A self with greater agency and freedom, one that answers less to parental phantoms of the past, becomes possible. It is in that sense, perhaps, that we can think of masochism as "a circle of freedom" (Butler, 1999, p. 147) (pp. 264-265).

This is provided clinicians are able to abandon countertransference issues that may lead them to pathologize perversions.

Hoff (2006), in her study involving four couples, discussed the idea of kink as a sexual orientation, an awareness of which can potentially come early in a person's life, comparable to homosexuality. While recognizing that not all BDSM participants have early fantasies or this early recognition, Hoff does point out that six of the eight participants in her study did, a notable number.

Gemberling, Cramer, and Miller (2015) also discussed the concept of BDSM as a sexual orientation, comparing it to the sexualities of lesbian, gay, and bisexual-identified people. To facilitate this comparison, the authors looked at sexual behavior, sexual attraction, and sexual identity. Then, within each of these areas, they compared and contrasted onset, consistency, and stability. One of the key findings was the difference that LGB individuals choose partners based on gender, while BDSM partners are chosen based on power dynamics.

> Therefore, expressions of a BDSM sexual orientation would revolve around a particular power dynamic: engaging in behaviors that generate a certain power dynamic, experiencing attraction towards acts with a certain power dynamic, and adopting an identity that conveys a certain power dynamic (p. 40).

Several authors have explored the idea of BDSM as a leisure activity, reconceptualizing the way in which theorists, clinicians, and those in academia have been taught to think of kinky sex, regardless of one's stance on psychopathology. Williams and Prior (2015) discuss about the spectrum of leisure activities, from casual to serious, speculating where BDSM might fall. In a study by the same authors, they found that kink shares a relationship with the characteristics of casual leisure:

> ...our findings suggest that BDSM participation may sometimes reflect qualities of casual leisure, such as playfulness, spontaneity, doing what comes natural, and childlike fun (Stebbins, 1997)" (Prior and Williams, 2015, p. 14).

Newmahr (2010) also makes the argument that BDSM transcends mere "kinky sex" and should be reframed as a leisure activity. However, she disagreed as to where BDSM falls on the leisure spectrum, finding that it has more elements in common with serious leisure, such as "effort, career, and durable benefits" (p. 6).

In a similar vein, Sagarin, Lee, and Klement, (2015) explored the similarities between BDSM activities and extreme rituals, such as body piercing, and found three main parallels. First, there was an increase in cortisol levels in both masochists and those undergoing piercings. However, simultaneously, the participants of both categories reported a decrease in psychological stress. The researchers attribute this to the second parallel, which was an altered state of consciousness.

> We assessed two altered states: flow (Csikszentmihalyi, 1991) and transient hypofrontality (Dietrich, 2003), which we believed might be the states described as topspace and subspace, respectively. Flow is a highly pleasurable and satisfying mental state involving intense absorption and optimal performance on an activity such as sports or music. In our studies, BDSM tops, ritual piercers, and those supporting a specific pierced ritual participant reported the highest levels of flow, particularly on the optimal performance facets of flow. Likewise, BDSM bottoms and non-piercer ritual participants (pierced participants, ritual leaders, drummers, observers, etc., but not piercers) showed decrements in performance on the cognitive Stroop test (MacLeod, 1991), suggesting temporary impairment of the brain's executive function capability consistent with subspace/ transient hypofrontality (Sagarin et al, 2015, p. 33).

The final parallel was intimacy. Beginning before the BDSM or ritual scene began until after it ended, the activities tended to bring participants together, whether or not there was sexual activity taking place (Sagarin et al., 2015).

GENDER ISSUES.

As I explored only the experiences of men, it was important to understand the stance of the literature on gender issues, particularly with regard to perversions and power dynamics. Freud (1905) stated that activity, a counterpart of sadism, was seen to be associated with masculinity, while passivity is associated with both masochism and femininity. This seems to fall in line with the stereotypical way that most boys and girls are socialized to behave. He later noted that femininity, and motherhood in particular, is actually quite active in nature. Benjamin (1998) followed up on this discussion, contradicting this view as a form of splitting. She instead proposed that a couple be seen as two subjects interacting *together* instead of a subject acting *on* an object, the latter of which merely acted as a container.

Yost (2007) researched the relationship between gender, sado-masochistic roles, and fantasies. She found that when BDSM practitioners identified with a stable role (Dominant or submissive), then gender is not a factor in fantasies. She notes that BDSM becomes "a place where stereotypical gender roles were reversed or outright rejected" (p. 149). However, for people who switch roles, the outcome is different. She theorizes that this may be because gender then becomes "more important as a guide"(p. 149) for expectations.

As stated earlier, Gemberling et al. (2015) compared the BDSM and LGB communities regarding sexual orientation. This also has implications for gender, too, however. The authors found that those identified as LGB based their sexual attraction, behavior, and orientation on *gender*, while those in the BDSM community based their sexual attraction, behavior, and orientation on *power dynamics*. This implies that the way in which we think of sexual orientation may need to be reconceptualized for BDSM practitioners at some point.

Countertransference reactions.

Countertransference is defined as "the whole of the analyst's unconscious reactions to the individual analysand–especially to the analysand's own transference" (Laplanche and Pontalis, 1973). This means that, though the analyst is mostly reacting to the patient's transference, reactions that are purely those of the analyst's also occur. When a patient discloses involvement in BDSM or having these types of fantasies, the personal feelings of the therapist may become involved and have an impact on the treatment.

De Peyer (2002) gives a clinical account of a patient (Richard) with sadomasochistic fantasies who came to treatment. She describes feeling oppressed and somewhat fearful of him in the beginning, though attracted to him as well. However, her fearfulness multiplied once he disclosed his sadomasochistic fantasies, with the desire for violence and murder to result, as well as his fear that it would. There was the added fact that he had, indeed, harmed someone years before while enacting part of this fantasy. The therapist describes her struggle with intense fear of Richard, though she fails to consider initially the implications of this countertransference reaction. She also discusses how Richard essentially dominates her for the first part of the therapy, while she helplessly submits. This eventually finds resolution once preoedipal issues begin to surface, and de Peyer's fear transforms to maternal empathy.

Richards (2003) pathologizes perversion by stating that she believes it to be "a source of pleasures that induce a person to devalue the pleasures of making love" (p. 2). She acknowledges that a certain amount of sadomasochistic behavior is present in all relationships. When detailing the three case examples that she puts forward, Richards makes the interesting observation that not only did these particular patients not come to therapy as the result of a perversion, but patients in general do not seek treatment for perversions "because perversions are behaviors that give them pleasure" (Richards, 2003, p. 3).

In a sociological paper, Nichols (2006) addresses the issues that may arise when patients report BDSM behavior to their therapists. One of the main themes focused on is countertransference and how negative feelings about BDSM practice may lead the therapist to focus on what are perceived as self-destructive behaviors. "When counselors find themselves believing that their clients' pathology is 'self-evident' despite no concrete evidence of harm, it is fairly certain that countertransference is present" (Nichols, 2006, p. 286) Additionally, Nichols (2006) states that this countertransference may be the therapist's "fears about their own 'darker' sexual desires" (p. 299). She discusses the various negative feelings that may be associated with acknowledging a facet of BDSM as a sexual identity and states that the therapist may reinforce a negative self-perception if an empathic response is not provided upon disclosure. Nichols goes on to compare the current state of BDSM in society to the place that homosexuality was in the 1970s, in terms of stigma. She advises to respect boundaries and not focus on the perversion if the patient has come to therapy for other reasons, unless the patient's sexuality becomes relevant during the course of treatment (Nichols, 2006).

Sociological perspectives on BDSM.

Weinberg (1995) works to dispel the myth that sadists merely seek to inflict pain and masochists to receive it. He cites Califia, herself involved in the BDSM community, who states that "the basic dynamic of S&M is the power dichotomy, not pain" (p. 291). The ideas of domination and submission appear to be the most important elements within the relationship. Weinberg (1995) explains that pain is merely one of many tools utilized by the sadist.

While this means that pain is not a necessary element, Weinberg (1995) asserts that the three essentials are control, trust and fantasy. He later expounded on these areas as key features of sadomasochism (Weinberg, 2006). First, the relational dynamic revolves around dominance and submission and not the pain that tends to be the focus of attention in mainstream society. Second, SM scenes are either scripted or have scripted elements and are meant to be enacted fantasies. There is an understanding between partners that the activities involved are role-play and not reality. Importantly, consent is a non-negotiable necessity between SM participants. While it is acceptable to enact coercion, it is prohibited by community norms to actually force an activity on someone.

Weinberg (2006) also states that sadomasochism is "symbolic," in that the assumed roles—either dominant or submissive—hold meaning for the person. Other meaningful aspects may include specific activities, manner of dress, honorifics, or implement utilized.

Simon (1996) cites Lotringer (1988), who says that "the purpose of the sadomasochistic contract is to make sure that power is never at stake. . . . The two configurations [dominant and submissive] overlap, both struggle to achieve separately their own singularity" (p. 22). Of the SM scene, Simon says:

> Actors are situated as an audience to the unfolding interaction; and, as such, they are split not only between activity and reflexivity but between identification with self and other as well. It may be that the lighting within the sexual chamber is dimmed, as often occurs, not to obscure what can be seen, but to see what is not present but must be seen (1996, p. 130).

Sisson (2007) states the evolution of SM over time shows that "an embryonic S/M sexual culture emerged in the late 1990s" (p. 157). This means that certain functions are performed by the SM community as a culture for its members, namely:

1. Demarcate boundaries;
2. provide a story of origin;
3. establish codes of behaviour;
4. create a system of shared meanings;
5. provide a means of social reproduction; and
6. generate sexual identity (p. 157).

The boundaries first mentioned help members decipher where it is safe to publicly acknowledge their sexual identity as being SM. Second, organizations, websites, books and participants preserve the historical facts that help to provide understanding to new members or others that might inquire into the culture. The National Leather Archives in Chicago are an example of how SM's history and story is kept intact by the culture.

Third, the culture establishes that participants will interact with each other in a certain way, relying on the edict "safe, sane and consensual" to guide activities. "Guidelines for S/M interactions, including preliminary negotiations about what will transpire, a 'safe word' which halts or slows S/M play, and 'aftercare' arrangements for monitoring participants' post-play reactions, are de rigueur" (Easton & Liszt, 2000 cited in Sisson, 2007; Wiseman, 1996 cited in Sisson, 2007). Fourth, SM participants share an understanding that the activities taking place are for specific purposes (sexual gratification, fantasy fulfillment, etc.) and are agreed upon by all parties involved. Fifth, communities have in place ways for new members to familiarize themselves with SM, the cultural norms, and issues such as safety. Meetings, or munches, are held where general information can be obtained, and safety demonstrations are also held in most communities or at conventions. Finally, all this helps the individual to establish his/her sexual identity (Sisson, 2007).

Currently, there are efforts by the SM community to have the Paraphilias section of the DSM removed. This is in response to clinicians diagnosing patients with Sadism or Masochism upon learning of consensual acts of SM, as well as the view by advocates that SM is not pathological (Kleinplatz and Moser, 2005; Moser and Kleinplatz, 2006; Langdridge and Baker, 2007). Reiersol and Skeid (2006) note that DenMark has already responded to these concerns by removing Sadomasochism from the country's ICD.

REPARATION

Laplanche and Pontalis (1973) defined reparation as the mechanism described by Melanie Klein whereby the subject seeks to repair the effects his destructive phantasies have had on his love-object" ("Reparation"). Klein (1935) theorized that the ego attempts to repair sadistic fantasies against the good object once the shift into the depressive position occurs.

The anxiety relating to the internalized mother who is felt to be injured, suffering, in danger of being annihilated or already annihilated and lost forever, leads to a stronger identification with the injured object. This identification reinforces both the drive to make reparation and the ego's attempts to inhibit aggressive impulses (Klein, 1952, "The Infantile Depressive Position," Section I).

Seen as a defense early in the depressive position, reparation serves to alleviate both guilt and anxiety resulting from aggressive impulses (Klein, 1952).

Reparative efforts begin during childhood and, if necessary, continue into adulthood with romantic relationships (Klein, 1964). Multiple attempts may be necessary for reparation to be achieved. Noting that parents are always psychologically involved in the selection of love objects, Klein (1964) states that, in relationships, we try to act as a good parent and a good child to that person. "In phantasy we re-create and enjoy the wished-for love and goodness of our parents. But to act as good parents towards other people may also be a way of dealing with the frustrations and sufferings of the past" (Klein, 1964, p. 67).

Weille (2002) asserted that there is a reparative element in sado-masochistic scenes with regard to earlier traumas or negative early object relationships. She details one particular case and walks the reader through the necessary elements of the relationship, including the "mind reading" of empathic attunement, the consensuality and the feeling of being safe. "Joan" describes how she has felt able to step out of her victim identity via SM and being in more of an active role in her daily life, as well as experiment with this sexually. The idea is that during scenes, she has a measure of control as to each act that is carried, as well as the result, which will not feel damaging to her this time. Rather, it keeps her in a position of power throughout, with Weille (2002) noting that there is no actual "subjugation."

Weille (2002) says that both Dom and sub are acting as containers for each other during the scene, with a loving and caring environment underlying an appearance of physical and sexual mastery and objectification. Also, "while sadomasochistic practices may diagnostically and etiologically conform with...psychoanalytic formulations, these same practices, under certain conditions, may also provide a means of working through the very developmental conflicts that gave rise to them in the first place" (p. 48). She states that the scene has to be "real enough" so that the person is put back into the same emotional place as during the original trauma, yet it cannot be so real that retraumatization occurs. Additionally, the relationship has to have a secure and loving foundation for these transformative effects to truly take place. Otherwise, the person may end up with repetition but no repair (Weille, 2002).

Bader (1993) discusses the fantasy and practice of sadomasochism as a way for dominant men to learn that their sexual power and desire can be welcomed, withstood and survived by their submissive partners. This works in the reverse as well for submissive women in their scenes with dominant men. His position is that these experiences function as a method of reassurance between the couple during the scene, and as a result, both people are able to fully enjoy the sexuality, aggression and power without the usual interference of guilt, concern for the other or self-consciousness about one's sexual force (Bader, 1993).

From a sociological perspective, Simon (1996) also notes guilt as one of three general themes of sadomasochism. A second is the repair of narcissistic pain, bringing forth a different type of reparative goal than that about which Klein (1952, 1964) writes. The prevention of fragmentation is the final theme.

IDENTIFICATION

The literature has shown that the multidimensional concept of identification has an important role in sadomasochism. Freud (1921) called identification "the original form of emotional tie with an object" ("VII. Identification," para. 7). According to Freud, identification involved the process of a child aligning himself with and internalizing characteristics of a parent in superego formation. In "Instincts and Their Vicissitudes," Freud (1915) discussed the idea of identification with the victim with the shift from sadism to masochism. Of this conversion and the relationship to pain, a theme in sexual sadomasochism, he states:

> When once feeling pains has become a masochistic aim, the sadistic aim of *causing* pains can arise also, retrogressively; for while these pains are being inflicted on other people, they are enjoyed masochistically by the subject through his identification of himself with the suffering object (Freud, 1915, "Instincts and Their Vicissitudes," para. 29).

This is also in line with the views of Ellis (1995), who, believing that sadists were concerned with the satisfaction of their masochist partners, stated that "it is highly probable that in some cases the sadist is really a disguised masochist and enjoys his victim's pain because he identifies himself with that pain" (p. 38).

Anna Freud (1936) later discussed the concept of identification with the aggressor as a defense in *The Ego and the Mechanisms of Defense*. She outlined two stages to this process. The first involves a role reversal with the aggressor, who is introjected, while the victimization is externally projected. Then, during the second stage, "aggressiveness [is] turned inwards and the entire relationship internalized" (Laplanche and Pontalis, 1973, "Identification with the Aggressor," para. 6). During a more recent panel discussion, Gillman also noted identification with the aggressor as a defense mechanism employed by sadists (Meyer and Levin, 1990).

Another view regarding identification in perversions comes from Glasser (1986). He makes the distinction between "identifying with" (temporary identification in which similarities with the object are evident) and "making an identification with" (a process in which permanent change occurs to the self-representation due to differences with the object). He contends that it is not possible for perverts to "make an identification with" an object, as this would be experienced or an invasion. Rather, he offers introjection as an alternative to the pervert being able to make identifications with objects. Through this process, "pseudo-identifications" are possible, which are referred to as "simulations" (Glasser, 1986).

There are multiple possibilities in this study for issues of identification to arise, whether it is identification with the victim, identification with the aggressor, or an inability to identify with one's partner at all, as Glasser (1986) suggests. Regardless, the literature indicates that identification plays a role in the relationships of sadomasochists.

EMPIRICAL STUDIES

Several studies have been conducted regarding BDSM in the fields of medicine, sexology, psychology and epidemiology. These serve to give an overview of what empirical data currently shows about this population in terms of their mental health and relational dynamics.

EPIDEMIOLOGY.

Richter et al. (2008) conducted a study in Australia, which tested three hypotheses about BDSM participants to see if they were:

1. More likely to have been victims of sexual coercion in the past;
2. more likely to have higher scores of on a psychological stress scale; and
3. more likely to have sexual difficulties.

They surveyed a sample of 10,173 men and 9,134 women via telephone, utilizing a computerized random-digit dialing system. There was an option to opt-out of answering BDSM questions if these made the respondent uncomfortable.

For both men and women, there were significant associations between engagement in BDSM and a higher number of lifetime sexual partners, as well as the gender of sex partners, meaning there was a higher likelihood of bisexual experiences. "Engagement in BDSM correlated strongly with a large number of sexual practice measures associated with greater sexual activity and interest in sex but weakly or not at all with the sexual history and pathological outcomes often assumed to be associated with 'sadomasochism'" (Richter et al., 2008, pp. 1664-1665).

The researchers reported no association between BDSM and sexual coercion before age 16; libido issues; orgasm difficulties; performance anxiety; sexual enjoyment; body issues; erectile dysfunction; or vaginal lubrication issues. "Men who had engaged in BDSM were significantly less likely to have elevated psychological distress, but there was no significant association for women" (Richter et al., 2008, p. 1663). None of the hypotheses were supported, and the researchers concluded that "BDSM is simply a sexual interest or subculture attractive to a minority, and that for most participants, BDSM activities are not a pathological symptom of past abuse or of difficulty with "normal" sex" (Richter et al., 2008, p. 1667).

SEXOLOGY.

Dancer, Kleinplatz et al. (2006) looked at lifestyle Dominant/submissive relationships in an effort to describe these 24/7 dynamics, as well as determine what differences exist between these relationships and those that consist only of bedroom role play or predetermined scenes. One hundred and forty-six submissives responded to an online questionnaire consisting of 49 questions exploring various aspects of the slave experience, such as rules, rituals, household responsibilities and relationship satisfaction. The sample consisted of 66 men and 80 women with a mean age 38. Forty-one percent were heterosexual, 26% were bisexual and 33% were homosexual. The median relationship duration was 24 months (Dancer et al., 2006).

The researchers had four key findings. First, in order to create and maintain a 24/7 relationship, "daily life must be structured by an unequal power differential" (Dancer et al., 2006, p. 93). While slaves did take care of many daily household tasks, there was a great deal of shared responsibility in lifestyle relationships. "There was little difference in tasks that are generally considered to be gender neutral (e.g., shipping, paying bills)" (Dancer et al., 2006, pg. 87). Rituals were reported by 86% (such as discipline or wearing a collar) and 99% had rules (Dancer et al., 2006).

Second, participants often had to engage in the power aspect of their relationship covertly. When questioned about being "out of role" while outside of the home, respondents described always functioning within the boundaries of their slave role but altering this in a way that works with the vanilla world (e.g., wearing a non-conspicuous collar, refraining from the use of honorifics). However, situations in which some respondents would be allowed to be "out of role" were sickness, when working or when with outside family members (Dancer et al., 2006).

Next, researchers found that safeguards existed to protect the slaves' safety, even though none of them had safewords. These included a discussion of limits at the beginning of the relationship, as well as the ability to stop a scene or, in 51% of participants, the ability to refuse an order. Even though many slaves stated that they gave their earnings to their Owner, the majority of slaves (60%) had bank accounts in their names. The significance of this is that they were able to access financial resources in order to leave the relationship should they choose to do so. Of the seventy slaves who had previously been in 24/7 arrangements, 48 ended these relationship themselves instead of the Owners taking this initiative (13 due to not feeling their limits were respected, having safety concerns or both). The researchers interpreted this as a sign that the freedom denied a slave during the relationship can be regained by the slave should she deem this necessary (Dancer et al., 2006).

Finally, Dancer et al. (2006) state that these 24/7 relationships mirror conventional relationship, in that within couples, standards of routine and acceptability are formed and the dishes need to be washed by someone. They found that slaves were treated as partners and not as the negative stereotype that is conjured when one thinks of and hears the word "slave." They note that 24/7 sadomasochistic relationships more closely mirror traditional marriages than they do domestic abuse situations (Dancer et al., 2006).

PSYCHOLOGY.

Cross and Matheson (2006) conducted three studies that they published in the same article regarding sadomasochism. The first study sought to test four academic views on sadomasochistic behavior: psychoanalytic, psychopathological, radical feminist and escape from self. Subjects were recruited via SM websites, as well as non-SM websites for comparison purposes (N=61). Of the 93 participants, 27 were sadists (21 men, 6 women); 34 were masochists (26 men, 8 women); and 32 were switches (22 men, 10 women). Numerous scales, as well as questionnaires created for the purpose of the research, were utilized to look at personality traits (psychopathology); sexual guilt and if sadists are driven by the id (psychoanalytic); feminist attitudes and attitudes toward women (radical feminist); and scales related to danger-seeking and role-playing (escape from self) (Cross and Matheson, 2006).

They found that significantly more sadomasochistically-oriented subjects reported being bisexual than the comparison group (sadists: 37%; masochists: 47.1%; switches: 67.7%; comparison: 18.1%). Also, SM participants were more likely to have had more sexual partners and to be in a stable relationship than the comparison group (Cross and Matheson, 2006).

With regard to the psychoanalytic perspective, Cross and Matheson (2006) found no association to suggest masochists feel sexually guilty or that sadists are id-driven. When they tested for psychopathology, the comparison group scored equal to or higher than the SM group on an Authoritarian scale. No other findings were significant for psychopathology. In terms of the radical feminism perspective, both SM respondents and the comparison group appeared to equally hold modern gender role ideas. Finally, masochists and switches were employed at a higher rate than sadists and the comparison group, who were employed at about the same rate. On a submissive scale, masochists and switches scored significantly higher than sadists and non-SM participants. There was nothing to suggest that masochists utilize SM or other behaviors as an escape (Cross and Matheson, 2006).

In their second study, Cross and Matheson (2006) looked at the differences between online sadomasochism and sadomasochism when practiced in person. A comparison group comprised of non-SM participants, including non-SM fantasy role-players, was utilized. Ten participants from the first study reported only engaging in SM online, so their responses were compared to ten randomly selected SM participants from the first study, as well as "Dungeons and Dragons" online gamers and non-SM participants. The Sexual Behavior Inventory, used also in the first study to discern sexual proclivities, was used here to determine appetites of virtual SM participants. Using cluster analyses, they first found that non-SM participants were in a separate cluster than SM participants, both real life and virtual. Second, they found that sadists, masochists and switches each formed their own clusters, though there was no differentiation between real life and virtual within the results. The grouping pattern was replicated in a second analysis with different samples (Cross and Matheson, 2006).

Their third and final study looked at the role of power in sadomasochistic relationships and questioned if pain is the goal of SM or merely a technique by which power is exchanged. Eight online couples were recruited and observed conducting scenes in online chat rooms. Interviews were then conducted with each person regarding the encounter, sadomasochism and demographic information. To evaluate power exchange, they looked at three factors:

1. The use of verbal or nonverbal cues or commands that guided the scene;

2. the exchange of personal information, signaling the lack of anonymity as a comfort; and

3. terms of endearment or expression of concern (Cross and Matheson, 2006).

Last, the researchers looked at how the power exchange was mutually created by looking for factors such as the use of honorifics, obedience, frequency of compliance with commands and checking in. They found that sadists were more likely than masochists to communicate their wants and needs directly, while masochists were more likely to either hint at their desires or utilize nonverbal communication. Sadists were significantly more likely than masochists to express caring or concern toward their partners. There were no significant findings related to the creation of the power exchange, as sadists and masochists were equally likely to utilize honorifics and check in with each other during a scene, even if this meant breaking role. Regarding pain, they noted that "we witnessed complex scenarios of submission and domination that seemed to use pain, if it was present at all, as more of a tool than a goal" (Cross and Matheson, 2006, p. 158). All of these findings give the reader an idea that BDSM relationships, particularly those centered on D/s, appear to be much more complex than the giving and receiving of physical pain. In fact, pain is merely a tool in the toolbox, so to speak. Rather, a more in-depth type of intimacy is hinted at from both Dominant and submissive.

Nordling et al. (2006) decided to look at a different aspect of BDSM culture, which dealt with the similarities and differences between gay and straight sadomasochists. A sample of 184 people (162 men and 22 women), all SM practitioners, was obtained from two clubs in Finland. They were interviewed via a mailed 237-item questionnaire. Due to the low number of female respondents, the researchers mainly reported on the men in the sample.

Nordling et al. (2006) stated their main finding as the emergence of a difference in the ways in which gay and straight SM participants engage with one another. They first found sadism associated more closely with men identified as gay and masochism more closely associated with straight men.

They then looked to see if there were differences between exclusively and predominately homosexual (n=90) and heterosexual (n=67) men and the ways in which they practiced SM. What they found was that gay men engaged in more activities geared toward hypermasculinity, while straight men engaged in humiliation play. Nordling et al. (2006) state that gay men showed a preference for "leather outfits, anal intercourse, rimming, dildos, wrestling, special equipment and uniform scenes" (p. 48), while straight men more often engaged in "verbal humiliation, mask and blindfold, gags, rubber outfits, cane whipping, vaginal intercourse, cross dressing, and straitjackets" (p. 48). The researchers also looked at possible childhood associations with the age the person first recognized their sexual orientation, both in terms of gender preference and SM interests, finding that gay men discovered their interest in and first experienced SM at a later age than straight men (Nordling et al., 2006).

Kolmes et al. (2006) explored the question of whether or not BDSM practitioners seeking mental health services had experienced difficulty in the therapeutic relationship as a result of disclosing their sexual practices. While they also had the intention of looking at the therapeutic interaction from the mental health practitioner's perspective, there was such a low response rate from therapists that they were unable to report on this.

Participants were recruited via an email announcement sent to various BDSM organizations, support groups and retail outlets, with 175 valid responses. Detailed demographics were taken, and of particular interest to this study: the state with the fourth largest number of respondents (11) was North Carolina; nearly ten percent (9.7%) lived in a rural area; and

35.4% stated one of their BDSM preferences as Domination/submission. Most participants reported only having seen between one and three therapists, and the vast majority (74.9%) went to therapy due to issues not related to BDSM. Most (65.1%) also disclosed their BDSM orientation with their therapist, even reporting they did this early in the relationship. Only 33.7% specifically looked for a therapist that identified as kink-aware.

According to Kolmes et al. (2006) there were a total of 118 instances of "biased" or "inadequate" mental health care that participants reported. They report the following six categories:

1. Considering BDSM to be unhealthy,
2. requiring a client to give up BDSM activity in order to continue in treatment,
3. confusing BDSM with abuse,
4. having to educate the therapist about BDSM,
5. assuming that BDSM interests are indicative of past family/spousal abuse and
6. therapists misrepresenting their expertise by stating that they are BDSM-positive when they are not actually knowledgeable about BDSM practices (Kolmes et al., 2006, p. 314).

More specific categories that participants reported as troubling were a lack of professional boundaries, feeling a duty toward mandated reporting due to BDSM activities, trying to specifically treat the client's BDSM lifestyle and "assuming that 'bottoms' are self-destructive" (Kolmes et al., 2006, p. 316). Participants reported 113 instances of positive experiences with therapists and also had the opportunity to give input regarding how therapists could be more kink-positive or become more kink-aware in a positive manner during interactions with BDSM clients (Kolmes et al., 2006).

The findings of these studies are relevant here in several ways. First, Richter et al. (2008) contradict the point of view held by many in the psychoanalytic field that BDSM is a pathological condition and normalizes it as a type of sexuality. Next, Dancer et al. (2006) were able to demonstrate not only a well defined structure to 24/7 BDSM relationships, but they were also able to show that these do not differ in major ways from the stereotypical traditional marriage. In vanilla relationships, each partner has the option to leave at any time, and this proved true in BDSM relationships as well, even with the female holding the title of "slave." This finding emphasizes the consensual nature of these relationships, which is a central concern to this study.

The most important finding from the Cross and Matheson (2006) study, for the purposes of this study, was that Dominants appear to hold feminist views outside of the scene. This contradicts the appearance of what their beliefs might be considering in-scene activity.

Homosexual and heterosexual BDSM are practiced in different ways, and this study helps to illustrate the reasons for not having a sample of both gay and straight BDSM practitioners for this study (Nordling et al., 2006). Kolmes et al. (2006) was able to show evidence of some of the difficulties that the BDSM population, and the participants, may have had with getting mental health help.

The South

As this study intends to sample from the rural South, it is necessary to consider what "rural" is, as well as what bearing the South may have on the data. The Census Bureau (1994) defines "rural" in the following way:

> Territory, population, and housing units that the Census Bureau does not classify as urban are classified as rural. For instance, a rural place is any incorporated place or CDP with fewer than 2,500 inhabitants that is located outside of a UA. A place is either entirely urban or entirely rural, except for those designated as an extended city.

According to the US Census Bureau, South Carolina has the thirteenth largest rural population nationally, with 39.5% of the state's inhabitants living outside of urban areas. This is 18.5% higher than the national rural population (SC Budget and Control Board, 2011).

There are three major themes of Southern life and history that have particular importance to this study. Religion, gender, and race all play significant roles in South, and interesting, all of them intertwine. Instead of separating them into their own categories, they will be discussed here in the interchangeable fashion in which they are lived, though all will be viewed from the lens of religion. "The Southern way of religion is different and has been on the most important and durable characteristics that sets Southerners apart in this nation" (Boles, 1999, p. 247).

Religion has been the cornerstone of many aspects of Southern life since the colonial years. Through two religious Great Awakenings, it was possible for Southerners to become spiritually independent from the Church of England. Throughout the second half of the 18th century, Presbyterians, Baptists, and Methodists formed individual denominations of evangelicism (Boles, 1999). Two of the basic guiding principles have been that each individual is both flawed – a sinner – and is responsible for their own salvation. Also, the way a person behaves directly impacts whether or not he will go to Heaven. Therefore, Protestants have always been focused on converting to the Christian faith in order to redeem oneself (Boles, 1999). Of Southern Protestant history, Boles (1999) states that:

> The focus on personal conversion was so all-consuming that Southern Protestantism was an intensely individualistic, privatistic faith. Certainly converts gathered together in warmly supportive church communities, but seldom did Southern white Christians conceive of their religion as having a social or reform dimension other than the reformation of individual sinners (which, it was believed, would translate into a better society) (p. 240).

While religion was a significant enough presence in the South for the moniker "The Bible Belt" to be bestowed upon the region, there were certain groups that were more "touched by the spirit" than others. Women far outnumbered men in church attendance as well as participation in church activities (Boles, 1999, Frazier, 2006). Boles (1999) gives a possible reason for this as women being grateful for finally having a definitive religious mandate against excessive alcohol consumption, infidelity, and other behaviors that interfered with the peacefulness and sanctity of the marriage. As only men were allowed to hold positions of authority in the church, it brought a new dimension to the argument for a man to tell another man he should not do certain things within his home and life. The power dynamic shifted somewhat, leaving men still in control, yet in a different way. Additionally, women now felt they had leverage against their husbands, reminding them of the danger their souls were in should they continue not living for the Lord (Boles, 1999). Frazier (2006) adds to this the important idea that, although women lived in an especially patriarchal society at this point, their involvement in church proved that there was one domain over which their husbands had no control: their salvation. The knowledge that only each individual could control this aspect of life may have provided some relief and agency for women.

While preachers felt comfortable delving into the personal lives of their congregations from the beginning, they did attempt to remain politically neutral for quite some time. However, as the Civil War approached and the North called slavery blasphemous, Southern preachers became defensive, both religiously and politically. After having been allowed to preach to black slaves and successfully converting them to Christianity, white preachers justified slavery as an ordinance from God. Along this same line of thought, losing the Civil War was offered as evidence that slaveholders were not Christian enough, and the loss was God's method of punishment (Boles, 1999).

At the beginning of this study, I recognized that the South's history of slavery presented a particularly interesting issue. I realized that there was the possibility of having a Caucasian participant who engaged in a consensual, sexual, Master-slave relationship with an African-American partner. Given the fact that any such participant(s) would have been raised in the South, the opportunity to learn more about their internal world during this type of play was an interesting prospect.

THEORETICAL FRAMEWORK

There were inherent drawbacks with making a definitive theoretical decision or constraining this study to one theory through which to see all data. It was important to not add to the preconceived notions that already existed. Therefore, it was the decision and goal of this study to allow the data to be naturally, organically seen through the proper lens as it was interpreted. The primary theory utilized was object relations, though there are some aspects of intersubjectivity and relational theory.

Object relations theory says that people, primarily caregivers, or characteristics of people are internalized. These internalizations help determine aspects of the personality, as well as interpersonal interactions (Klein, 1935; Fairbairn, 1952). Contemporary theory adds that the maternal object's engagement with and responsiveness to the infant are especially important (Elliot, 1995). There are two states of intrapsychic being: paranoid-schizoid and depressive. When in the paranoid-schizoid position, the person is guarded and fearful of the harm that may come from external objects, referred to as annihilation anxiety. When in the depressive position, the focus of the anxiety shifts to the fear of doing harm to others.

Winnicott (1969) contributed the complex idea of object usage to object-relations theory. Here, he said that what occurs is a multiphase process. First, the subject begins to relate to the object. Winnicott differentiated object usage from object relating by noting that relating involved the use of projections, while object usage does not. When using the object, the subject seeks to destroy the object and appreciates the object's survival. Winnicott (1969) describes this process by way of the following:

> The subject says to the object: "I destroyed you," and the object is there to receive the communication. From now on the subject says:

"Hullo object!" "I destroyed you." "I love you." "You have value for me because of your survival of my destruction of you." "While I am loving you I am all the time destroying you in (unconscious) fantasy." Here fantasy begins for the individual. The subject can now use the object that has survived (p. 713).

This destruction is not borne of aggression or the wish to exploit the object. In fact, object usage means that the subject has relinquished the fantasy of omnipotent control and recognizes and appreciates the object's autonomy. Additionally, Winnicott (1969) notes that it is only considered destruction if the object does not survive, which is then the object's failure, not the subject's. What constitutes survival is the object's ability to continue the relationship with the subject without a "change in quality or attitude . . . it does not retaliate" (Posner, Glickman, Taylor, Canfield, & Cyr, 2001).

One important aspect of this concept is that Winnicott (1969) believed this process of destruction/survival occurred in fantasy. Ghent (1990), when applying the idea of object usage to surrender, postulated that the failure of the object to survive destruction as described by Winnicott would ultimately result in sadism.

RESEARCH QUESTION.

What does it mean to be a heterosexual male Dominant in the rural South?

Related questions:

1. What is the quality of their relationships with significant objects?
2. Were there any traumatic events that occurred before adulthood?
3. Has their sexual identity affected any religious ideals or other values that may have been instilled in them as children?
4. Has the subject experienced discrimination based on his sexual identity?

DEFINITIONS OF MAJOR CONCEPTS.

Dominant: "One who enjoys performing any of a variety of BDSM practices upon a submissive; or one who holds a dominant position within a relationship based upon dominance and submission [D/s]." A male dominant is referred to as a Dom, while a female is a Domme (both have the same pronunciation) (BDSM Terms and Definitions, section "D," para. 10).

Limit: A stated boundary with regard to an activity, which can be verbal, psychological, sexual or physical.

Restitution: For the purposes of this study, restitution will be defined as the process of working through, understanding, and/or finding meaning in an experience or internal conflict. This will also include Stoller's (1991) concept and process of the transformation of passive into active.

Rural: For the purposes of this study, an area will be considered rural if its population is less than 30,000, according to the Census Bureau data available for the period of time during which the participant lived in that area as a child.

Safeword: A predetermined word or set of words used by the submissive to either slow down or completely stop an activity if necessary. If gags or other impediments to speech are being used, gestures replace the spoken words (BDSM Dictionary, Section S).

Scene: The play, sometimes prearranged roleplay, that takes place between submissive/bottom and Dominant/Top (BDSM Dictionary, Section S).

Submissive: The person in a D/s relationship who "yield[s] to the control or power of another" by consensually giving up their own control (BDSM Dictionary, Section S).

Vanilla: A person who does not engage in BDSM activities (BDSM Dictionary, Section V).

ASSUMPTIONS

This study made the following assumptions about the area of inquiry:

1. Where there is sadism (domination), masochism (submission) will also be found.

2. The BDSM culture is not based in aggression but is rather constructed around concepts of equality and consensuality cloaked in psychodramas of inequality.

3. Dominants raised in the South will have likely been raised with Judeo-Christian beliefs and, as such, may have internalized a sense of guilt about their sexual identity, practices, and/or fantasies.

CHAPTER 3

METHODOLOGY

STUDY DESIGN

The population studied was a combination of two groups that have both, in their own right, been largely neglected by the research community, as the South's sexual practices have been little studied and the BDSM community as a whole has been shied away from by many researchers. As such, there is no existing information specifically regarding the experiences of BDSM Dominants or sadists in the South. Therefore, this study was exploratory and qualitative in nature, utilizing a case study approach, as employed by Tolleson (1996).

In using this approach, a small sample is recruited, and a series of in-depth interviews then conducted with each person. The purpose is to seek deeper meaning from a small group of individuals regarding their experiences as expressed by them. Data from each individual case is analyzed separately and a cross-case analysis is completed, in which common themes are discussed (Tolleson, 1996).

Runyon (1982) stated that three of several goals that the case study method can accomplished are: "Helping us understand the inner or subjective world of the person, how they think about their own experience, situation, problems, life. . . . Deepening our sympathy or empathy for the subject. . . . . [and] Effectively portraying the social and historical that the person is living in" (p. 152). These were salient issues for this project and in line with the goal of finding deeper meaning regarding the phenomenon.

In the original study, seven participants were interviewed. Yin (2009) notes that, with multiple-case studies, "typical criteria regarding sample size . . . are irrelevant" (p. 58), and that the number of cases will reflect "the number of case replications—both literal and theoretical—that you need or would like to have" (p. 58). He continues that a higher number of cases, "five, six, or more replications" (p. 58), are desirable when the theory involved might be more implicit than explicit or when additional certainty is preferred (Yin, 2009). For the purposes of the original study, it was felt that at least seven cases would provide sufficient replication, a high level of confidence in the data, and lend ample opportunity to strengthen theory.

While seven participants were included in this study, two made the decision not to be included in this publication. Therefore, the focus will be only on the remaining five, as the results did not undergo drastic changes and maintained their integrity.

SCOPE OF STUDY, SETTING, POPULATION AND SAMPLING, SOURCES AND NATURE OF DATA.

For this study, each participant was interviewed five times each. The criteria for study inclusion were as follows:

- Male
- Sexually identifies as a Dominant
- Heterosexual
- Age 25-59, the largest age categories for BDSM practitioners (Brame, 2000)

- Either raised in the rural South or has lived in the rural South since latency
- Currently lives in the South
- Must be either in a relationship or has had prior D/s relationships. This was to ensure that the participant had transitioned from fantasizing about BDSM activities to actually engaging in them.

I initially contacted BDSM organizations by email in both rural and more metropolitan areas, with nearby outlying rural areas, within North and South Carolina, in order to seek subjects for recruitment into the study. However, I never received a response. I then utilized a popular BDSM online community, reaching out to group leaders through this medium. After receiving permission to advertise, I then proceeded to recruit participants from local organizations via this online community.

If interested in participating, the potential subject contacted me, and a prescreening interview took place via Skype to see if all inclusion criteria were met. Data collection interviews then took place in the subject's home. Due to the distance involved in traveling to some participants, Skype was utilized to assist in conducting interviews.

DATA COLLECTION METHODS AND INSTRUMENTS

Semi-structured interviews conducted with research subjects were the study's main source of data. The first interview was utilized to gain an understanding into the participant's childhood experiences and life. Subsequent interviews related to the subject's sexuality, relationships, and internal and relational experiences during a scene.

At the beginning of each interview, each subject was reminded that he had the option to stop at any point during either the day's interview or the series of interviews. They were also reminded of their confidentiality throughout the process.

As interviews were the method by which data was collected, the researcher was the primary instrument for collecting the data. All interviews were recorded and transcribed. Field notes were also made during each interview to help capture detailed nuances that did not translate to the recording, as well as my own reactions to the participants and data. Additionally, these field notes will serve to begin to identify patterns across cases.

DATA ANALYSIS

The case study analysis looked at each person's unique experience of being a Dominant; events in their lives that may have shaped their sexuality; the psychological function and importance of BDSM for the Dominant; and the ways in which they view themselves and interact with others.

As interviews were taking place, there was a continuous awareness of themes, patterns, and meanings that were emerging. Once all interviews were completed, individual cases analyses as well as a cross-case analysis were conducted (Tolleson, 1996). First, each individual case was analyzed, which involved coding the participant's interview transcripts, and listening for categories of meaning to emerge from the data. Then, a cross-case report was completed, in which all cases were analyzed for unifying themes. Yin (2009) notes that conducting a cross-case synthesis adds robustness to a study of this type and strengthens the findings, as well as any resulting explanations or theory.

By using an interpretive lens that is psychoanalytically focused, this allowed for the consideration of not only the data collected from the participant but also my own interview reactions as well. Loewenberg (1988) states that "the acceptance and utilization of countertransference as a tool of insight in clinical practice and research is the most important post-Freudian development in the theory of technique in the past three decades. . . . Today, the countertransference is an appropriate part of any case report" (p. 145). Though these reactions were not true countertransference, as they did not occur within a clinical situation or a therapeutic relationship, the nature of the reactions occurred in the same spirit. It is in this vein that my interview reactions were interpreted and utilized as a form of data. As a way to control for internal validity, the researcher kept a journal during data collection of personal thoughts and reactions. Also, one member of the dissertation committee was utilized to discuss various interpretations with as a way of ensuring against researcher bias (Tolleson, 1996).

PROTECTING THE RIGHTS OF HUMAN SUBJECTS

Participants were assigned an identification number as a way of safeguarding their true identity. Interviews were conducted in environments where the subjects could feel assured of his privacy, in all cases, the participant's home. All data collection materials, such as tapes, transcriptions, and field notes, will be kept by the researcher in a locked box to ensure confidentiality. The data will be retained for five years.

At the beginning of the first interview, I presented each participant with an informed consent form. The form was discussed in detail and did not proceed until comprehension was evident. Each participant was encouraged to ask questions or express concerns then, as well as at any point during the process. They were also informed that they had the option to withdraw from the study at any time and were asked if they wanted to continue at the beginning of each interview.

Chapter 4

Findings

What follows are the case studies for each of the five participants who chose to have their stories told here. They include the participant's family background, relationship history, BDSM history, unique categories of meaning, and my interview reactions to the participant. All names have been changed. Notably, participants #1, 2, and 3 chose their pseudonyms, while the remaining two did not.

Participant 1: Falcor

Falcor is a 46-year-old, divorced, heterosexual Caucasian man, who lives in North Carolina. He is tall with an athletic build and engages in several different sports. Falcor has a Master's degree in the humanities, though he works fulltime in the business world. He described an active social life, enjoying frequent engagements with a wide circle of friends.

At the time of the interviews, Falcor was living with his fiancée, whom he married the following year. He seemed eager about his participation, though he disclosed that his partner had vetted the project online, verifying the legitimacy of the study, before he became involved. Notably, she was also present for the prescreening interview and greeted me when I arrived at their home for the first interview. He also checked with her before scheduling subsequent interviews to get her approval regarding times and dates.

At each interview, Falcor seemed relaxed, friendly, and enthusiastic. He was usually dressed in casual clothes, sometimes as if he was about to work out. For the in-person interviews, he always offered me a drink, both alcoholic and non-alcoholic. He drank some type of alcoholic drink in most of the interviews, usually wine, though he never appeared intoxicated.

Family history.
Falcor was born in Arkansas and raised there until age four. He then moved with his family to an urban area of North Carolina until he was 10 years old. At that point, they moved within North Carolina, returning to a rural area, where Falcor remained until high school graduation.

Falcor is the middle child of three boys. When discussing his parents' relationship, he described his father as "dominant" and his mother as "very subservient." He expressed clear disagreement with the way in which his mother was treated, noting that his father would "yell" at her. The discipline in the home was meted out by his father.

> He had a weird concept that, almost like when you train a dog. You hit 'em right away when they do something wrong, immediate correction. Correct the problem right away by being physical. He'd hit us, slap us, punch us, if we did something.

Falcor's mother died in the mid-'90s in a motor vehicle accident. She had raised the children in the Catholic Church and was "the glue that held the family together." Her death was devastating for Falcor, who was particularly close to her. After her death, he stopped going to church and became agnostic, which is his current religious identification. His father was also critically injured in the accident but made a full recovery.

Four months later, his father remarried. At the time of the interviews, the relationship between Falcor and his father had healed to the point where they were able to get along well.

Falcor is not close to his older brother and referred to him as "creepy." Interestingly, this brother also identifies a Dominant. However, Falcor expressed that he and his brother have differing philosophical views regarding BDSM. He seemed uncomfortable talking about him, and when I asked him about this, he was only able to explain it by his brother's characteristic of being "creepy."

He is close with his younger brother, who is a minister. Falcor noted ironically that his brother has an addiction to pornography, which allowed him to feel comfortable disclosing his sexual identity to him. Despite his brother's religious affiliation and career, their shared appreciation for sexuality that is considered by many to be taboo provided an avenue for further bonding.

While growing up, his father was relatively liberal regarding sex, as he lived abroad for a period of time. However, his mother did not discuss sex. He felt that he father would be accepting of his involvement in the BDSM lifestyle if he were to disclose this, but he had not shared this information with his father. His mother also never knew, and he made it clear that he never would have told her.

Significant relationships.
Falcor has been married and divorced twice. His first marriage was with his college sweetheart at 23 years old. He described them as having been great friends who enjoyed playing various sports together, but who should not have gotten married. Falcor and his first wife remained married for 11 years. She was quite religious, and, according to him, "asexual." He notes that they did not consummate their marriage on their wedding night. During the course of their marriage, they had sex a handful of times each year, and Falcor describes going through elaborate romantic rituals to ensure that the experience was pleasurable for her.

This included making sure their young child was out of the house, lighting candles, giving her a massage "for an hour or two," and performing oral sex. "It'd take two or three hours to where she really, really wanted to have sex." After his mother's death, he began having affairs, which was a contributing factor in their divorce.

Falcor's second marriage was to a woman who was much more sexually adventurous. She was a Dominatrix by profession, though submissive in the marriage, and they agreed to allow swinging in their relationship. As such, they established a sexual relationship with another married couple: Falcor's fiancée and her then-husband. However, his wife and the other husband in the arrangement ended up falling in love with each other. Falcor and his partner then began dating, and each couple divorced. His second marriage lasted four years.

Falcor and his fiancée had been together for two years when I interviewed him. They were planning their wedding for the following year, which I later learned did take place. Falcor expressed a great deal of hope that this marriage would prove successful. "You know, she and I have both been married twice and – failures. You know, we're gonna do it again. Third time's a charm – I think it will be. Cause, God, we really love each other."

BDSM background.
Falcor first became interested in BDSM when he was 14 years old. He recalled seeing a magazine that featured fetish material in it and found it arousing. However, he described himself as a "late bloomer" and an "awkward" teenager, so he did not have the opportunity to experiment until later. During his first marriage, he became bored with mainstream pornography and found a BDSM film which featured a rape scene. This was exciting to him, though his wife found the tape and degraded him for his interest.

After his mother died, Falcor had his first BDSM experience. He began having an affair with two women, who were a couple. Both were looking for a male Dominant, and Falcor began having sex with them and learning about BDSM. After his divorce, he had multiple casual relationships with women who were submissives.

He identifies his main kinks as rape scenes and bondage, while his hard limits are guns and blood. He does not consider himself to be a sadist and described pain as "a tool to heighten her awareness, to change her state of consciousness." He is actively involved in his local community and, therefore, many of his friends are aware of his sexual identification as a Dominant.

CATEGORIES OF MEANING.

BDSM as a form of play.

Falcor is very specific throughout the interview process that his Dominant persona is very separate and distinct from "Steve," his given name. He describes Steve as being "loving" with his partner, both in and out of the bedroom, viewing her as an equal. Falcor, however, is:

> totally different. . . . He doesn't make love; he fucks the hell out of her, among other things. I think she needs that, and I need that, too, you know, and the things that Falcor does to her are [things] loving Steve, the husband-to-be, can't do to her. And I need love in my life. My Dom personality doesn't have that in him – it really works for us to have that split personality.

He described their BDSM play as an escape. When asked the reason for the escape, he responded:

> Because I guess the real world just doesn't, I mean, you can be happy in the real world, but I think it helps us especially when we were, you know, she was a troubled teenager. I was a pretty happy teenager overall, but it's always helped us escape, and we both have very vivid imaginations. And the creativity that BDSM brings is a great outlet. I think a true BDSM Dom is like an artist.

The canvas is your sub, and you're creating something beautiful
with the scene.

This allows him to play various roles in "a total fantasy world." Here,
he is able to safely explore fantasies for which he has been criticized in the
past. He and his partner have acted out rape fantasies, slave auctions, and
brandings, all within the confines of pre-determined limits. Of the faux
branding they enacted, Falcor said that "had that not been negotiated in
a lot of communication and it had not been somebody who we have such
a close relationship with, I couldn't have ever done that." At one point,
Falcor compared it to when he played Dungeons and Dragons as a child:

> I used to be the dungeon master, and I felt that my responsibility
> as a dungeon master was to make sure all my players, four to five
> people in my world, had a good time. And I think I want her to
> have a good time. I want her to have a fulfilling experience and
> usually have a lot of orgasms, but she doesn't necessarily have to,
> I suppose, but it has to be something they enjoy.

Entering the fantasy world of BDSM allows Falcor respite from the
difficulties of daily life. He is careful with his own limits to keep the
real world from seeping into his refuge. Falcor is clear that he does not
engage in age play of any kind because he has a daughter of his own. He
acknowledges that this is too close to reality for him to gain any type
of pleasure. Also, he emphasized several times that during their rape
scenes, it is important that she not struggle too much.

> I don't want to have to really hurt to control her. And it's, you
> know, I don't know how real rapists actually get a hard-on, if it's,
> because it's so intense. If you're doing such physical exertion,
> even though I'm a pretty strong guy, I work out all the time, if
> you have to play that part to control somebody, you're not gonna
> get a hard-on right away unless you use overwhelming brute
> force. Punching. And then you're talking about breaking bones
> and knocking somebody out, or using a knife. And then if they're
> fighting really hard and you've got a knife, that can be dangerous.

During such a powerful scene, he is careful to set the condition that it not be too realistic. If it becomes too realistic, then it no longer qualifies as play. In these instances – age play and rape scenes – the scene becoming life-like would breach boundaries and create anxiety which Falcor is aware he would not be able to tolerate. Part of the reason for this may be the element of reenactment that is occurring. During a scene, he allows himself to become physical and theatrically brutal, which is reminiscent of the genuine manner in which his father behaved. Falcor is able to experience this and enjoy a temporary identification with his father, provided he feels comfortable and remains within the agreed upon limits. However, if part of the scene feels too real, then that would strengthen Falcor's feeling of similarity to his father, which would eliminate any conscious pleasurable aspects for him.

In addition to the fantasy aspect of the various scenes, there is also the contrasting reality of how their relationship actually functions, which indicates that BDSM truly is play for them. Several times, Falcor expressed concern about ensuring that there is balance and equality between them. He recognizes that during a scene, they play at inequality, but that it is important for the health of the relationship for that to end with the scene.

> I don't want me to be above her. I want us to be equal, you know, and that feels good to me, you know, I open her doors for her. I told you about that. And I think domming her 24/7 . . . I've never been . . . attracted to women who really wanted that, you know, that wanted to . . . have their life totally controlled.

The BDSM scene as restitution.
Falcor was able to clearly identify power and control as aspects of the scene that he enjoys and actively feels at the time. This is evidenced by the types of play in which he engages as well. In addition to rape scenes, Falcor describes other scenarios that put him in a powerful position. He stated that a typical scene may start with him texting her during the day with "sexual innuendos to...start the foreplay even before she comes [home]." He then described buying her as a slave at an auction:

> I'll look at her, I'll go up there and smell her hair and say how pleased her Master is with her appearance, how her legs are looking, how she's dressed. I'll rub up against her, and then I'll beat her in there, I'll sometimes say, well, I'm going to test your mettle today. I'm going to test how much pain you can take, see if you are worthy of, you know, Master Falcor's cock.

He later elaborated about this particular type of scenario.

> Eighty percent of the time, it's me initiating it, but when we're playing in that role, she's to beg for me to fuck her, to even let her see my cock or suck it or hold it. I like it when I make her do the cock worship thing.

Falcor described himself as a "late bloomer," noting that in high school he was not found attractive by girls. The experience of having a woman beg for him sexually, worship his genitalia, and be able to deny her or make her wait for a length of time to be determined by him is not only incredibly powerful for him. It also functions as restitutive to those narcissistic injuries from adolescence.

> Growing up, like I said, kind of a late bloomer, so, yeah, it was mostly us guys trying to chase the women. So when you learn to reverse that . . . as a Dom, and have women chase you and then actually beg for you, that's a pretty powerful thing. And so that's the big turn-on for me.

Additionally, Falcor not only gets to have power over his partner, but he is able to have a certain amount of dominance with other men as well. If other men want to play with her, then he is the gatekeeper for this and makes the decision as to whether or not this is acceptable. He also protects her from other Doms who may try to cross boundaries. He described a playful wrestling scenario between his partner and another submissive that became more serious when another Dom became involved.

He said to her "I'm going to make you submit." And I had to have a talk with him. I said, "You're not going to. You need to clear that with me." He actually started crying. I didn't try to make him cry or anything. I was just trying to educate him going forward.

Here, he was able to show not only that his partner is "his" and protect her, which in itself is restitutive for him, but he was also able to inflict humiliation on another man. Protectiveness plays an important role in Falcor's history, as he was unable to protect his mother from both his father and the accident which took her life. With his partner, he is able to keep her safe from other Doms, which are unknown variables, as he does not know the full extent of the harm they are capable of causing her, though he may unconsciously fear that, just as with his mother, this may mean death. Also, in his own play with her, he keeps her safe from any harm he fears he could do, by way of his own control. These protective actions are likely restitutive for him, as he can feel certain he is protecting his partner in the ways he was not able to protect his mother.

Therefore, when he fails at this type of control, it will remind him of his own vulnerability and fallibility. When discussing what his responsibilities are during a scene, Falcor said:

Well, safety for one thing, make sure they don't get hurt, that you don't violate any of their hard limits because that would destroy the trust. . . . [E]specially when you're dealing with knives, I just make sure I don't go too far. You never want to lose control. You never want to get so turned on that you step over a line. You never want to play inebriated. We drink every day, but I never play drunk. That's the main thing. You make sure you're sound and well rested because it doesn't work if you're tired. It's too much of a responsibility.

He also noted that his partner has only used her safeword twice: once, so that he could learn her limits and the second time due to unexpected pain. He acknowledged that he felt guilty and reinforced that he is not a sadist. However, when allowing her to play with someone else, she was burned with the wax from a black candle.

> [The person controlling the scene] gave me a black candle, and it kind of burned her skin a little bit with the candle wax, and it's still got little marks from that. Tiny little marks on her back – that makes me feel a little bit weird that I left a lasting mark with candle wax. [I feel] a little guilty that I didn't protect her. I didn't intend to leave a mark, and there it is. So it's a mistake I made. I feel a little bit guilty about that, and I'm going to make sure it doesn't happen again. I look at her back today, and there they are a constant reminder that I screwed up one time.

Falcor's demeanor here changed. He became solemn, quiet, and his voice was heavy with responsibility. He clearly felt that he failed in his job of protecting her, and any positive psychological effect that may have come from that scene was lost when she was hurt. He is reminded of it when he sees the mark and masochistically continues to blame himself, even though he was not the one in charge of the scene at the time.

BDSM as a means of connection.
Falcor frequently talked about the connection that he felt with his partner both during and after a scene. This was one aspect of their quality time together as a couple. "There's a fulfillment that you focused on one thing – that's the scene – and that can be pretty amazing when, suddenly, the world is pulling you different ways. To take two hours just totally devoted to each other in a scene."

He consistently reminded me of the amount of trust that she must have for him in order for their interactions to happen at all, and he seemed in awe of that at times. "I feel a lot of love that she would, you know, trust— she would allow me to [be dominant with her]. I think that strengthened our relationship in other ways."

Aftercare seemed to be an area that also strengthened and solidified the connection between Falcor and his partner. After a scene is over,

Falcor said that his day-to-day persona returns for aftercare. He explained the purposes of aftercare:

> To show her she's loved, you know, and appreciated and trying to bring her level of anxiety – her heart rate down. Her heart is beating a lot after, you know. Trying to comfort, trying to get her to feel loved and trying – re-establish more of a loving connection, more of almost an equal partnership because, first, we're not really married and then that's . . . wanting that to be an equal fulfilling partnership for both of us. And aftercare brings that back. Afterwards, we're an equal couple again. So in a scene, I'm the dominant. She does whatever I tell her to. She better do it right then. So total power exchange. It just brings it back to normal. We're not 24/7 Master/slave; we don't want to be.

When Falcor talked about the various emotions that he worked to ensure his partner experienced during aftercare, it can be imagined that he feels those same emotions as well. He says that:

> I think just the emotional, the love, afterwards. She's very, very needy afterwards. She needs to be cuddled, and I love that, love holding her. I mean, I love just cuddling with her, but, to me, the aftercare brings everything full circle. I couldn't ever imagine not doing it.

One of the purposes that aftercare served for Falcor was that it gave him the opportunity to see that she survived the scene, still loved him and was willing to accept love from him. The brutality of his alter ego did not destroy her or their relationship.

INTERVIEW REACTIONS.

When I initially pre-screened Falcor, he seemed very friendly and outgoing. In fact, he suggested that I go out to dinner with him and his partner at some point, and I wondered if he would be able to respect the boundaries of the researcher/participant relationship. However, upon meeting him I quickly saw that he was respectful, even a gentleman. I was struck by his appearance and, admittedly, sexually attracted to him.

I noticed that he seemed to need additional time with me after the interviews, especially the ones that took place in person. He would walk me out to my car, and we would talk for another ten to fifteen minutes. I realize that this was a different version of the connection that seems to occur during aftercare. The interviews were intense and thought-provoking for Falcor. He mentioned he had not experienced having someone listen to him in this way before (not a dialogue *about* but rather an inquiry *into* his experiences). Therefore, to leave abruptly at the end of the interview would have broken that connection off too suddenly. It was the functional equivalent of providing aftercare for him.

Falcor did find it difficult for the interviews to come to an end, and in my own reaction, I also had a hard time letting go for fear of inflicting some sort of emotional damage. This was a clear signal as to how fragile he actually was and how fearful he likely was of losing those in his life, especially his partner. I realized towards the end of the interviews that I had begun to associate to a small golden Labrador puppy anytime that I thought of him, an association that continues today. This seems to fit with my impression of and reactions to Falcor: friendly yet vulnerable.

PARTICIPANT 2: BOB

Bob is a 59-year-old, separated, Caucasian male, who resides in South Carolina. He lives alone in a duplex, which he rents, and is retired from the manufacturing business. He referenced his adult children throughout the interview process, and has frequent interactions with them. Bob seemed to be somewhat socially isolated, saying that he has been called "antisocial" in the past, though he disagrees with this assessment.

All five interviews were conducted with Bob in person due to his location. At each interview, it was noted that he was dressed in motorcycle gear, and he acknowledged a love of riding. Bob's home was always neat, and his two cats remained close to him throughout each interview. Bob generally was able to talk about BDSM with ease, though it became slightly more difficult for him to describe his emotions related to the scene as we progressed to the later interviews.

Family history.

Bob was born in a relatively urban area of Iowa and spent the first three years of his life there. When he was three, his father received a job transfer, and the family moved to a very rural part of South Carolina. Bob continues to live in the same town today.

Bob's mother stayed at home taking care of the three children. He described her as "crazy" and "an abuser." Bob was open in talking about the fact that she was both verbally and physically abusive to his brother, as well as his feelings that this was wrong. He also talked about the fear that witnessing this abuse created, saying that it "...did strange things in my head. Like, if she can do that to him, you know, I could be next."

Bob also described his mother as a "pet serial killer." He explained that she became known throughout the family for quickly growing tired of caring for pets and having them put to sleep. Bob stated that he, too, felt callous toward animals for a long time and expressed remorse for the way he used to treat them. He gave the example of hunting as evidence of his former maltreatment.

Bob's father also worked in manufacturing. He was gone much of the day and was required to work some nights and weekends as well. Bob seemed to have conflicted feelings toward his father. He described him at one point as wearing the pants in the family, yet he also stated that "Dad was kind of like water and electricity; he took the path of least resistance. So, he pretty much did whatever mom wanted to do." His father died ten years ago, and it was only at his funeral, when he heard another family member question why his father had never intervened on his brother's behalf during the childhood abuse, that Bob says this thought first occurred to him. He has concluded that, while his father may have turned a blind eye to some of his mother's behavior, she was "smart enough" to hide most of the abusive activity from him. He also gives his father credit for occasionally stepping in to defend them as children.

Bob grew up with two older siblings, a brother and a sister. His brother died of cancer in 2007, while his sister continues to live near him, and they see each other on occasion. When Bob was growing up, he recalled that his parents' attitude toward sex was that it "didn't exist...just a great unmentionable." It simply was not a subject that was ever discussed with him until after he was a married adult. Bob learned about sex from "peers, dirty books, and experimentation," as well as from the standard health class in school. He stated that he doubts his father would have cared had he been aware that Bob was involved in BDSM. However, he feels his mother's reaction might be different and joked that perhaps he should tell her.

Significant relationships.

At 18 years old, Bob met and married his wife. They have been married for 40 years, though are now separated. The reason he gave for this is that "I was tired of her breathing my air." Within their first year of marriage, his wife had an affair, with which Bob struggled. He expressed feeling that she told him about it as a way to relieve her own guilt.

Later, he had an affair, of which he said his wife was aware, that lasted 20 years. He described this woman as an alcoholic who, at times, had difficulty controlling her temper. She would also call his wife to tell her about the relationship and taunt her with this information. The affair ultimately ended because of a difference in expectations, her behavior, and her alcoholism.

Bob has three adult children – two daughters and one son. He described having good relationships and frequent contact with them. All of them live in the same area as Bob, and he visits with them as their schedules allow. Bob said that at least one of his children is aware of his involvement in BDSM, though this does not bother him. He explained that, while he does not subject them to information about his personal life, he also makes no effort to conceal who he is.

BDSM history.

Bob began engaging in BDSM soon after he started having sex. He described kinky sex as being something which he and his estranged wife both enjoyed. However, when they first got married and began experimenting with BDSM, they did not realize that it existed as an organized sexual identity or community.

> I didn't know it as [BDSM] then, but I just knew that we were always looking for something to push the envelope, take it a little higher or make it more exciting. And it would start out...buying fancy lingerie, and then it would escalate. Bondage and some light BDSM-like whips or something like that. It just didn't dawn on me though it was BDSM. It was just trying to find something fun to do behind, you know, closed doors in your own bedroom.

Since being separated, Bob plays with various submissives that he meets online. He considers these women to be his friends, though he does not speak of their interactions in terms of committed relationships. He is not involved in the local community at all beyond its online presence.

Bob identifies his main kink as "messing with people's minds" or, in community vernacular, the "mindfuck."

CATEGORIES OF MEANING.

BDSM as restitution.

> Maybe [the BDSM scene is] reminiscent of the way my mother used to abuse my brother. Maybe I'm just dealing with Mom's abuse or something, I don't know. My way of preventing myself from going and choking the shit out of her. Exacting revenge. Maybe my way of reconciling that. Maybe that's the underlying

reason that I like it...It probably empowers me, and there's so
many aspects of life – everyone does feel powerless and helpless
and at other people's mercy.

Bob was placed in a position of helplessness and powerlessness as a
child at the hands of his mother, particularly watching as his brother was
abused. He was open in expressing his disdain for his mother and her
actions, as well as acknowledging that this had a profound and lasting
psychological impact. He also talked about his father's either inability
or unwillingness to protect them from their mother, though it was more
difficult for him to talk about this, and he appeared more defensive and
comfortable with excusing his father's inaction. Bob also addressed his
own inability to help his brother at times when he would witness the
abuse. It is likely that, along with the hatred for his mother and guilt
for his helplessness, came an admiration and desire for the power and
control that she wielded on a daily basis.

During a scene, Bob is able to take his former helplessness and convert
it into empowerment by virtue of his ability to feel in control. "I like
being in control...that's probably a big part of it." Through his present-
day control in the scene, he has found a safe way to give expression to the
pain of the past. It is essentially a method of showing another person the
raw images of hurt that words may sometimes elude. Additionally, Bob
noted several times that "...when I'm in control, the sub is in control." He
is aware that the scene is co-managed by both partners in a shared power
dynamic. This means that, unlike his siblings and him, the submissive is
able to stop at any point for any reason, revealing her true power in the
situation. It is important to realize that this plays with the same type of
dynamic which existed between his parents when he was a child. There
is the illusion of the male holding all of the power, though the female
of the dyad has the ultimate power.

For Bob, BDSM scenes follow a much different emotional script. Not
only is he able to feel the elusive and sought-after control, he is also
able to please the submissive.

> If I wanted to please or serve this sub, I would do anything I could
> to that end. My behavior is driven by the sub. It makes me feel like
> I'm good for something. Gives me purpose, because eventually,
> if I fulfill [her needs], she'll fulfill mine.

In Bob's re-creation, he is able to know what is required of him through predefined parameters, adhere to those, and feel certain that he is working toward gaining the submissive's approval. He receives confirmation of this when she consents to sex in the later part of the scene. When this happens, he experiences a certain amount of reciprocity. While this appears to be orchestrated rather than genuine, Bob experiences it as his needs being met.

This approval he receives from the submissive is important because Bob is clear that he has never been able to receive approval from his mother. He mentions her negativity throughout the interview process, as well as the value she places on material possessions instead of people.

In the scene, the approval and acceptance of the sub provides a momentary but satisfactory substitute for the approval Bob never received from his mother. During aftercare, Bob works to confirm this approval in what he jokingly calls a "post-game interview." He checks with the submissive, questioning her about what they have just experienced together, to ensure that he did meet her expectations and has gained her approval.

Bob was careful to note that he does not enjoy engaging in dangerous or risky types of play nor does he want to actually hurt the submissive. He discussed the fact that he recently went beyond his own comfort level in order to provide for the submissive the level of satisfaction she sought. Bob had difficulty connecting affect to this experience, saying "Maybe I'm just short-circuiting my emotions or something." One is left to wonder if he fully achieves from the scene what he desires in a situation in which he feels he has crossed his own limits or if his goal of "serving the submissive" mitigates this.

The Dom role as a safe exploration of aggression.

> It's not hard to get into the role for me because I suppose it's like an actor playing Hitler; if you really thought you were Hitler, you might go hang yourself. But you've got to keep your eye on the fact that you're an actor portraying somebody else, for the entertainment of somebody else.

During the scene, Bob is able to step out of his usual state of helplessness and self-described depression and experience a version of the power he has witnessed his mother utilize throughout the years. He expressed his feelings about the concept of power, saying "I don't particularly enjoy power, sadism, but I like to play." Bob seems to utilize the familiarity he has with his mother's aggression, as well as emotional manipulation, for the purpose of the scene. In an ironic tone, he refers to it as an "opportunity to use all the skills I saw my mother use so well."

However, Bob is able to recognize that if he too closely identified with her during the scene, then he would feel transformed into the person he hates, overwhelming him. Therefore, by choosing the path of BDSM, he can be certain that his partner is consenting to the actions taking place and, therefore, that he is not being abusive, as was his mother. The brevity of the scene also allows for the exploration to view in the context of the role of an actor, so that he can reassure himself that he has not absorbed this aspect of his mother's personality on a permanent basis.

Bob talked about the experience of being in this position of power. He stated that "it's a good feeling to know that you can make them do anything you want," though he handles that "as responsibly as I can." One aspect of that for him is checking in with the submissive throughout the scene.

> Even during the scene, a lot of times, I'll stop. Take a break and ask 'em, "Do you know the safeword?" Because you get so fucked up on that shit, you might not even remember, or you might not even be able to talk. So, it's important to keep a finger on that particular pulse and make sure that she's not so far out there,

you go too far. I could hurt her, and she might be incapable of saying the safeword. And I might cross a limit and basically, if you do that, you don't really have their consent. You've just set up a condition where she's incapable of giving consent.

Clearly, while Bob enjoys being able to explore his aggressive side, he also seems to make a distinct effort to ensure that joint control of the scene is maintained. If the submissive becomes too caught up in the scene, is unable to verbalize the safeword, then that leaves Bob continuing to enact this aggression against a person whom he no longer feels is consenting. In that scenario, he would likely feel as if he, too, was an abuser, like his mother. "I don't want to abuse the person. And abuse, defined for me, is crossing her limits."

These limits are also an area with which he takes a great deal of precaution. He requests that potential submissives respond to a 200-300 item list, detailing to which activities they do and do not consent.

It helps me to put it down in black and white, so at least I have some kind of plan. I'll end up with a list saying that these are things she likes. These are kind of things that are on her edge, and these are things that are strictly off limits. So that just keeps me from wandering into bad territory for them...As long as I stay within the boundaries of the list, I should be in fairly safe territory.

While "in character" during a scene, Bob stated that he feels he has "kind of a license to mess with people's minds" and this is part of what he enjoys. "I like playing on their fears." When this is successful, he acknowledged that this is part of the "payoff" for him. Here, Bob has the opportunity to take the emotional manipulation that he saw inflicted by his mother and play with it. He can manipulate the situation and the person, be dishonest, and create discomfort. There is also the element of physical pain, which he states he applies carefully.

BDSM as a safe emotional connection.

> "The stronger the activity, it could be argued that it makes stronger bonds, and it's not much stronger activity between two people than having sex – unless it's kinky sex."

As Bob explores his aggression and achieves restitution by obtaining the submissive's approval, then he is able to receive "the final payoff," which he talks about in terms of sex. However, he alluded to a deeper level of fulfillment beyond the physical. "It's just a warmth towards that person, a connection with them, and a feeling of being needed. Useful." Several times, Bob refers to the interaction of the scene as "serving the sub." When asked to elaborate on his use of this, he says: "Because they have the safeword, they're really in control, actually... they're calling the shots, and I just think, from my perspective, a good Dom is wanting to make himself aware of the sub's needs and serve them."

The connection that Bob feels is more firmly solidified during the process of aftercare. Bob described aftercare as:

> Lots of touching, cuddling, vanilla sex, as much as possible. I like to spend the night with them. That way, we can just sit there and spoon them all night if you want to. That could evolve into more sex, even if it is vanilla. So, that's part of my payback, part of my payoff. And, you know, once you've done a scene with somebody, it kind of breaks down a big barrier, and afterwards, people [are] probably a little more open with each other. It also gives me a chance to see more of the real them.

His use here of the word "payback" and frequent use of the word "payoff" during our interviews validates his idea that, during the scene, his actions are driven by what the submissive wants from him.

Bob went on to here to talk about the deeper connection he feels with someone with whom he has engaged in a scene. Given his admitted propensity to "shut his emotions off," I wondered if the openness he referenced was a pleasant experience for him or if it felt uncomfortable and he was merely going through the expected motions.

> No, it's good to feel it. I mean, maybe that's what I'm seeking. Maybe that's another one of my big payoffs. It's a connection. I've always had problems relating to people, and this is one avenue that I can relate to people.

Not only Bob's mother but also his estranged wife and former lover have shown him that it can be dangerous to get too close to women. On the surface, he speaks of sex as being his "payoff," though it seems as though he uses physical intimacy as a mechanism for seeking the possibility of an emotional attachment. At the least, he is able to experience momentary closeness. Bob identifies as monogamous "95% of the time" and states that he "detests quickies" because they are "too damn animal" for him. He utilizes the BDSM scene as a way of feeling he has control of the situation, and then it likely feels much safer to approach the submissive on an emotional level. His statements about monogamy and "quickies" do present an interesting paradox, however, as he had a long-term affair within his marriage and BDSM can certainly be categorized as aggressive play, even animalistic. There seemed to be certain aspects of himself that were difficult for Bob to acknowledge at various parts of the interview process.

BDSM sex and aftercare as validations of aggression survival.
Though Bob was superficially nonchalant during the interviews about his identity and role as a Dominant, he made statements to the contrary. For example, throughout the process, he made a point of reinforcing that he does not enjoy the infliction of pain, is not a sadist, has negative feelings towards sadists, and that he cares about the physical and emotional wellbeing of his submissives. It seemed important to Bob to emphasize his differences from that of a sadist, as he likely considers his mother. This is also why he may consider animalistic sex to be unacceptable. Any association with his mother is likely to be something which he

finds repulsive and from which he works to distance himself. He views "quickies" as aggressive, the main quality of his mother, and therefore finds it to be an unacceptable part of his life.

He referred to sex at the end of a scene as his "payoff" multiple times. When he described the post-scene activity, and into aftercare, he depicted a great deal of affection that takes place. Beyond the physical, Bob seems to be in a state of relief. He has enacted this aggression, which he links to his mother and has been reliving to play out. The sex is then evidence that she was able to survive his aggression, a reward for controlling himself and not fully identifying with his mother. The sex, then, is also the comfort that he likely feels he needs after this type of reenactment.

During aftercare, he checks with her about how the scene felt for her, did anything go wrong, what he did right, etc. He seeks detailed feedback so that he can ensure that she did, in fact, survive and no harm was done. He needs this reassurance from his partner that consent was present throughout, that he did fulfill her desires, and that he did not achieve a complete identification with his mother. Should the submissive seem uncertain after a scene, sustain injury, or express negativity (such as anger) towards him, any positive effects of the scene would also vanish for him.

INTERVIEW REACTIONS.

When I first met Bob, it felt hard to connect with him. He seemed friendly enough but guarded, and I worried about whether or not he would feel comfortable enough to open up to me during the interview process. Additionally, his description of himself as having been cruel to animals was difficult for me to hear, and I felt judgmental of him. It was only as I watched him with his cats and saw his genuine affection toward them that I was able to remind myself that this had merely been one additional area of life which his abusive childhood had affected.

As we progressed through the second interview, I began to get the feeling that he was lonely in his solitude. Also, I realized that I was still not entirely comfortable around him. I felt relieved when I left and worried that I had rushed through the first two interviews, though I later realized that I had not. This was a reflection on the discomfort that he still felt by allowing someone into his personal space, which was confirmed in the final interview when asking him about his thoughts on the interview process.

Q: Has it been weird or uncomfortable?

A: No. Once I got over the fact that I let you in the house.

As we moved into the middle of the interview process with the third and fourth interviews, I noticed that he and I had both begun to relax. As our discussions centered on BDSM, Bob seemed able to talk more openly and deeply about his experiences, particularly in the fourth interview. I could feel that he had settled into the rhythm of the process and was at ease with it. Toward the end of the fourth interview, he was able to finish a couple of my questions for me. I felt a great deal of empathy for his childhood struggles, and I noticed that I was careful to avoid issues that might cause him to feel discomfort or emotional pain. Was this a genuine reaction or my internal IRB committee member cautioning me? Perhaps these were simultaneous processes which occurred. However, I am more inclined to believe that there was an unconscious collusion taking place. As I look back on it, there seemed to be a moving away from and reluctance to deepening the interview in certain moments to avoid hurting or reinjuring him in response to an unconscious plea. This is certainly evidence of his continued vulnerability, as well as a connection that formed during our time together.

Bob also seemed to enjoy very brief conversation after the recorder was turned off. I did not sense that he wanted this to be prolonged, and he made no move to continue the conversation beyond its natural ending point or keep me longer. He was always very polite, walking me to the door, and usually holding it open for me. He always cautioned me to watch my step carefully as I exited his home. During these times, I felt as though he was being protective in a kind, almost paternal, manner.

I ended the interview process feeling still more guarded with Bob than with other participants, yet connected to him on a certain level. I felt myself looking beyond the asocial personality that he presented and feeling warm toward the underlying person who struggled to form safe attachments with others.

PARTICIPANT 3: MR. R

Mr. R is a 49-year-old, divorced Caucasian male, who lives in North Carolina with his female partner of two years. He currently attends college, working toward a degree in the mental health field. Mr. R and his girlfriend are active socially, particularly within the BDSM community, attending various events and parties. They live in a quiet, suburban neighborhood and appeared at ease interacting with each other.

Mr. R is friendly, though guarded in many of his responses throughout the interview process. It appears difficult for him to talk in great detail about his own emotional responses to situations, and he had to be pressed to deepen and elaborate on these answers much of the time. He seemed much more at ease discussing his partners and their reactions, though it is possible this was a function of projection, given his historical BDSM journey.

Family history.
Mr. R was raised in a military family and lived many different places for the first several years of his life, including the Philippines. His father served three tours of duty in Vietnam, and Mr. R recalled the difficulty of those days:

> There was no more terrifying sight to a child or a wife of a military service member than to see an official sedan drive up the

street. That memory is indelible because every kid knew, to see two uniformed men in a car driving **up** your street meant that somebody was dead or badly injured or missing, and whatever prayers that people say at that time, you know, you just – "Dear God, don't let it stop at my house."

After Vietnam, his family settled in a rural area of Florida, which was almost entirely comprised of a military base. Mr. R lived there with his parents and sister, two years younger than him, from age eight until he was 18.

His parents had traditional gender roles. However, his mother was responsible for the daily operations of the house and family during his father's war service. Mr. R described his mother as "independent" and spoke of her with admiration. He stated that she made the decision to trade a career as a successful corporate executive, unusual for a woman at the time, in order to become a military wife and mother.

While he recalled that his parents presented a united front regarding family issues and decisions, he was aware of "discord."

> There was some conflict in my family concerning me, in particular. Dad didn't have a lot of good parenting skills, he was trying to mirror the parenting skills that he saw which were horrible; he had a very dysfunctional family. He wanted the best for me, and he was very supportive of me, but he was also very demanding and he was a very directive parent. "Do this" instead of explaining this, so he wasn't a good teacher. So that made a big difference, and I'm pretty stubborn, so we butted heads quite a bit.

However, he said that there was very little corporal punishment used in his family, though when there was, it was "ritualized."

> "Get. The belt." It was none of the "Wait until your father gets home." Mom would sometimes break out the wooden spoon, too. But dad had actually a particular belt that was in the closet and, you know, "Get. The belt." But I really can't think of any more than a handful of times, especially in my preteen years, I was punished.

> By and large, the punishment, discipline in my home was tempered with as much of trying to understand why something was being done and why it was wrong as it was anything else.

His father was also an alcoholic, who drank for all of Mr. R's childhood, though later became sober once his health began to deteriorate. He died in 2007.

Mr. R's mother left the marriage after 30 years, once both he and his sister were adults. Mr. R stated that she "just couldn't do it anymore," referring to his father's alcoholism. He described remaining relatively close with her after the divorce, though he notes he was not close with his family of origin in a traditional sense once moving out after high school. His mother passed away as a result of cancer four months prior to the start of our interviews.

Mr. R's sister lives in the Midwest, and he has no contact with her. He stated that he "never particularly liked" her.

> In many ways, we are diametrically opposed in pretty much everything. She is very happy to be told how to think, what to do, where to go. And I just, I don't have a lot to say to her. But I wish her well, you know. May the gods keep and protect you, far away from me.

Mr. R stated that he was aware of the presence of sexuality in his house as a child. His father had "erotica" hung in the bedroom as part of the décor, and also had "a lifetime subscription to *Playboy*." He recalled hearing "obvious signs and sounds of sex" as well while his parents were married. However, he viewed his mother differently.

> You know, mom might have been pretty asexual. Hell, she might have been even a lesbian for all I know because it was never a subject of discussion. I never saw her express any interest with dating or going out and meeting men after she left dad. I never saw any sign that my mother was sexual. Never found any dildos, vibrators, anything like that.

Significant relationships.

Mr. R has been married three times. He married his first wife while he was in college, and this marriage lasted five years. They experimented with some BDSM activity toward the end of their marriage, with the sexual roles being "fluid." They also engaged in polyamory. Unrelated to this, Mr. R stated that she decided to leave the marriage for one of his best friends.

His second wife, to whom he was married eight years, was diagnosed with "rapid-cycling bipolar with homicidal and suicidal tendencies." During this marriage, Mr. R helped raise two step-children and said that feeling a responsibility toward them was the reason that he remained in the marriage as long as he did. This relationship did not have a BDSM component and, in fact, was not very sexual, especially for the last two years. Upon separating, he discovered that she had been poisoning his food, which accounted for some health issues which he had been experiencing.

His last marriage lasted only two years, and Mr. R describes her as "jealous." He states that she was constantly concerned about his fidelity, and this, along with her depression, led to the downfall of their relationship. She was in the BDSM community and worked professionally as a Dominatrix, while being submissive to Mr. R.

He has been in his currently relationship for two years and states that they have no plans to marry for financial reasons. He describes her as being different from his other partners in that she is independent, financially secure, and emotionally stable. They do engage in BDSM, and he states that she is "owned property." By this, he says that he means they consider themselves to be "Master" and "slave," though "the terms are mutable."

BDSM history.

Mr. R states that he had an interest in his father's erotica, which showcased some BDSM. He also once experimented with it as a young teenager, tying up a girl from his neighborhood. Mr. R first explored his interest in BDSM as an adult during his first marriage, though this relationship was mostly vanilla. Also, he initially explored the role of submissive. After his divorce, he continued to participate in BDSM, though acknowledges that he "got in over [his] head immediately." Mr. R entered an abusive relationship with a female Dominant, who others in the community helped him leave.

During the next five years, he explored switching between dominance and submission in his relationships. He described experiencing a great deal of personal growth and healing during this time. He then made the transition to the identification of Dominant, which he called "an evolution," saying "I had explored as much as I think I could, at that point."

Mr. R identified his main kink as the power exchange and noted that he is "a pretty healthy sadist."

Categories of meaning.

BDSM as a compromise formation.

> "If I don't have a submissive who's willing to give me trust, then what am I? I'm just a guy with a bag of toys. I'm just an asshole who's an abuser, bottom line."

Mr. R's first experience with BDSM was tying up a girl of the same age as a young teenager.

> A: She didn't resist when I tied her up and had her on the bed in my bedroom. I realized I was about to break a whole bunch of laws and get myself into trouble, and I kind of freaked out and came to my senses.

> Q: In what way were you about to break a whole bunch of laws?

A: I think she was probably about to get raped

He continued talking about this experience, stating that he was afraid of getting caught by his parents and their reactions, particularly that of his mother. He categorized it as "a wakeup call."

> Oh, my goodness, I don't want to do anything that I don't really plan to do and have control over. So, I didn't really like that feeling of being out of control. I was aware of what I was doing was, you know, had some negative connotations. Mostly, I couldn't believe that I had almost done that.

Feeling the urge to rape her had a powerful impact on him. He realized that he had nearly lost control of himself and did not enjoy that lack of control. Additionally, he feared the legal, practical, and parental consequences of being caught. However, this does not necessary negate the desire he initially experienced to exercise power and control over a partner; he exercises control over the impulses in order to avoid societal sanctions which would otherwise be imposed.

Through the compromise formation, Mr. R seems to have defensively transformed these desires, channeling them via the practice of BDSM. Though BDSM is by no means mainstream, it is arguably more tolerable to the general public than sexual assault. His participation in BDSM allows Mr. R to enjoy the feeling and experience of controlling a woman and having power over her while having the crucial element of consent. This way, he is relieved of any potential guilt while also avoiding practical, i.e., legal ramifications.

However, these desires continue to be evident in his play. Mr. R does engage in rape scenes, which allow him to consensually act out and participate in those fantasies. He also participates in "take down" scenes, in which physical dominance is exerted to overpower the submissive. Mr. R acknowledged that on one occasion, he has "violated some limits."

> Primarily because the relationship I was in, I was getting such mixed messages on the limit that I chose to violate it. It was anal play. And there was, you know, the young woman had been anally raped. She was clearly asking to safely explore it at the same time while stating it was a hard limit. There was a lot of "Oh, that looks so good, I'd like to feel that. Don't ever do that to me." Yeah, so, I, you know, I didn't. One night I had her in scene, I had her bound, and then we started going there.

Mr. R appeared able to utilize BDSM in its various forms to transform his desire for power and control over his partners through the use of the compromise formation in the vast majority of instances. However, it seems that this defense does fail him when presented with a situation where he feels confused, frustrated, or not in control of the situation, such as by being presented with undesirable limits.

BDSM also provides Mr. R with an acceptable outlet for his sadism. When he talked about scenes in which he is able to fulfill sadistic desires, he described a reciprocal relationship. "I was giving her something she needed. At the same time, I'm getting fed by it because I'm getting to hurt a pretty girl." When describing how it feels at the time to hurt her, Mr. R took a deep breath and said "It feels like ambrosia."

There is a significant difference between how he feels when inflicting pain and when he has control.

> If somebody wants to voluntarily let me whale on them until they are screaming, crying, and jumping around, that's fun for me because they've consensually allowed it. I'm generally never sexually aroused. It turns me on, but, I don't, you know, I've never had a raging hard on from beating somebody. The control aspects turn me on; the sadistic aspects are just fun.

Dominance as a restitutive defense against powerlessness.
Mr. R experienced many things in his childhood over which he had no control: moving to a foreign country; his father serving in Vietnam and

the constant fear that they would be notified of his death; practicing "duck and cover" drills at school; an alcoholic father; and family dynamics that evoked a power struggle between himself and his father, of which he was on the losing end. As an adult, he endured an abusive relationship in which he had no control and "was being micromanaged" in a "very, very strict" environment. He survived a marriage during which his wife attempted to murder him.

His response to this overwhelming powerlessness has been a transition to a situation in which he has total control. In the interviews, he was even unable to verbalize the word "limits" when discussing his partner's significant health issues which do prevent them from engaging in certain forms of play.

> A: I would say it's a "no limits" relationship, other than the limits I impose on it.
>
> Q: But it sounds like, you know, that she has limits, health issues, for example, and that you are respecting those limits, even if y'all don't call them that.
>
> A: Yeah, we talk, we communicate very well. We talk a lot, you know?
>
> Q: But aren't those limits?
>
> A: (hesitates) They are areas of concern.

Having control in this relationship helps him to defend against the vulnerability that he has experienced in previous relationships and situations. To consciously acknowledge that there are limitations beyond his control, at least in this manner, would be threatening to him and expose that vulnerability.

Mr. R is comfortable acknowledging that "bottoms hold the power." However, this seems to only be in the larger scope of referring to BDSM as play and to submission as a gift instead of the narrower context of his own relationship. As long as he maintains dominance in the relationship, then he feels he is limiting his risk of exposure to the variables which have caused him suffering in the past.

BDSM as a connection.

Both in casual scenes and within his relationship, Mr. R stated that he has to feel a connection to the person. Otherwise, he does not continue with the scene. "I've stopped scenes because the connection wasn't there. If it's not working, it's not working." He elaborated with a story of a seasoned masochist who was receiving birthday spankings from different people at a party. When he hit her, she responded with the challenge "Is that all you got?" Mr. R disengaged and walked away. "If you are so jaded, if you are not connected, you're wasting my time. My energy is too precious to give to you."

From that connection, Mr. R expressed feeling fed "emotionally, energetically, even intellectually."

You're creating a moment. In some ways this is some of the most intimate behavior that humans can engage in. Somebody has allowed you into their personal space, you'd let them use their flesh as a canvas, has allowed you to create all of these emotions and feelings and experiences together.

Along with that connection is a desire Mr. R has to address the needs of the submissive, whether this is his partner or someone in a casual scene. "After the safety issue, then my responsibility is to create an environment, the moment, that is nurturing and fulfilling for both of us." This extends into aftercare, which Mr. R describes from his perspective:

> You know, I am a nurturer, and I do enjoy that intimacy because the aftercare moves from a particularly intense scene where the bottom has really gone someplace special for them. We continue to have that moment. It's kind of like drifting on a lake a night, a

warm southern night. It just kind of surrounds you in this glow. We're continuing to share whatever we created

INTERVIEW REACTIONS.

During my meetings with Mr. R, he was friendly, personable, and I generally enjoyed interviewing him. His length of time in the community, and particularly his experiences as a submissive made him unique. I both appreciated that and was intrigued by it.

I noticed right away that he seemed to have difficulty connecting affect with the events and situations he described. This continued throughout the interview process. There are multiple reasons that he may have been guarded in this manner (personality, unfamiliarity with me, caution due to the profession he plans to enter, etc.). Regardless of the reason, I felt as though I had to work especially hard to engage in the process as compared to other participants. During the first interview, there was also a distracting factor for me. We met in the kitchen and sat at the table across from each other. Behind him, in a mail holder that was facing me, was a very small flogger. It seemed out of place, as there were no other toys visible in the area, and I found myself wondering if it had been intentionally put there, for looks or to garner a reaction of some sort.

Mr. R seemed to relax marginally as we moved through the interview process, and this seemed to help me relax as well. At the end of our third interview, as we moved toward the door, Mr. R expressed a concern that those who would read and evaluate this project – at the time, my dissertation committee – would be unable to understand fully the nature of BDSM because they would, presumably, be vanilla. I was startled and felt myself becoming defensive; after all, I chose the members of my committee. I assured him of my committee's professional knowledge, experience, and capabilities, and he seemed to accept this.

During the interviews which were conducted in person, Mr. R seemed to enjoy a brief amount of talking while I was gathering my materials and re-packing them. This was also about the same for the Skype interviews. He did not seem to need a great deal of post-interview care from me.

PARTICIPANT 4: TOM

Tom is a 40-year-old single Caucasian male. He lives with his girlfriend and their infant. Tom works in the IT field and is employed by the family business. He also provides child care for his son during the day while working from his home office. He and his partner have been together for four years and are moderately active in the BDSM community. Tom is tall, slightly overweight, and a calm, easygoing demeanor.

During the interview process, I met with Tom at his house for all but one interview, which was conducted through Skype. He seemed relaxed and forthcoming, able to talk with relative ease. During our fourth interview, when privacy was a concern because his partner was home, our interview took place in the basement, where Tom has play equipment set up that he, his partner and a select group of friends occasionally use.

Family history.
Tom was raised in a rural area of South Carolina, where he continues to live.

Tom's family consists of his mother, father, and a brother five years younger than him. His parents are still married but live separately now with no plans to divorce. During their time living together, the relationship was contentious, and Tom recalls arguments between them. He noted that his mother was particularly apt to argue, and his father was better at controlling his temper.

Tom's relationships with his family are relatively good. He gets along well with both parents, though he sees his mother more than his father by virtue of the fact that they do business together. As a child, he recalled power struggles with them.

At about 10 years old, I was having issues in one of my classes, and the teacher was like "He's not doing his homework." So, they started taking stuff away from me to try to get me to do my homework, and it got to the point that my room was an empty room with a mattress. And I still wouldn't do whatever they wanted me to do. And Dad and I sat down and talked, and he pretty much figured at that point that I was going to do whatever I wanted to do.

This carried over into other aspects of life. Also at 10 years old, his mother began to work more, and he "became a latchkey kid" and was home alone after school. "But, I mean, at that stage, I was already enough of my own person that I could do that anyway." As a teenager, his parents left it up to him to decide whether or not to continue going to church.

Tom states that he is sometimes "irritated" with his brother, and appears slightly annoyed by the fact that he continues to live with their mother. "He's a little cocky and full of himself sometimes, and he thinks a lot more highly of what he thinks he knows than he should."

During Tom's childhood, his father worked various jobs, changing jobs frequently at certain points. When he was in second grade, the family moved multiple times. Tom does not recall the reasons for this, stating, "all I remember was changing schools a lot." At one point during this period of time, Tom and his family lived briefly with his grandparents, both of whom are now deceased. He also spent time with them throughout the year. He described their marriage as being one with traditional gender roles, typical of their generation and era.

When asked about his parents' attitudes toward sex, Tom stated that "there was no discussion of it. At all." However, his grandparents "were very open about stuff, where other people weren't. And I mean, nowadays, it would not surprise me, if it [had] existed then, that they would have been in a BDSM group or a swingers group." He recalled seeing pornographic magazines in their house, as well as finding erotic cartoons that his grandfather had created.

Significant Relationships.

Though Tom has had many relationships, he has never been either married or engaged. He has had several long-term relationships, all of which had a BDSM component to them. "I never really tried vanilla relationships...It just doesn't feel right to me." One of these relationships lasted for eight years. He stated that, though it began as a power exchange relationship, the dynamic shifted to vanilla over time. Tom initially left after four years, only to return when his then-girlfriend threatened suicide. After six years, he discussed with her that he was unhappy and needed things to be different between them. Two years later, the relationship ended.

Another of Tom's relationships began as a power exchange, evolved to vanilla, and ended after two years. He categorized this former girlfriend, who also made threats of suicide, as "borderline insane." However, because she had physical health issues, she continued living with Tom for an additional two years. During this time, she had surgery, and Tom assisted "somewhat" in her recovery.

Tom has been with his current girlfriend for four years. This relationship also began with a power exchange component. "Currently, it's not functioning that way. We've got to work on getting that back into the relationship again, but, you know, with [a baby], things kind of went to hell." When asked if he tends to be attracted to chaotic women, he responded:

> I don't know if I'm attracted to them, but I end up with them. That might be my subconscious working, I don't know. I tend to be attracted to stronger women. Women that are gonna – not just be that total doormat mentality, and so, in that case, I might be picking people that are gonna be a problem.

BDSM history.

"I enjoyed tying girls up when I was little, and I didn't even understand what the heck it was." Tom recalled being interested in aspects of BDSM as a young child, tying up other children during games, such as cowboys and Indians, and enjoying that. Once he began interacting with girls, this activity escalated. "My girlfriends, by the time I was 12, if they did something I didn't like, I would turn them over my knee and spank them." However, he acknowledged that he was unable to fully comprehend the meaning of this action at such a young age.

Tom said that he has always known that he desired BDSM relationships and never considered an alternative. In addition, he stated that he has never experienced any guilt about this. His family is aware of his sexual identification.

Tom follows a particular sect of BDSM known as Gor, which is based on a series of science fiction novels that began in the 1960s. The Gor books reference Master/slave relationships, though Tom acknowledged that it is still grounded in and under the umbrella of Dominance/submission. He explained the philosophy as follows:

> In [the Gor] books...females are predominately submissive. That's where you end up with the quotes like "A woman is never totally free until she's a slave" and things like that. There's a lot of philosophy through the books, and it's like, yeah, that makes a lot of sense. Because to an actual slave, when they become a slave is when they can really be them, and that's a form of freedom. It's the same for the masters, you know. Until we are allowed to live our lifestyle, we don't really feel free because we're constantly fighting who we are. I mean, if that's who you are, then denying [that] is just going to lead to conflict.

In line with his relationship philosophy, Tom stated his main kink as "control," the power exchange. In terms of activity, he prefers bondage.

Dominance as a compromise formation.

Tom describes having anger issues as a child. "I had an extraordinarily bad temper when I was younger, but I learned to control it and channel it." He gives two examples of this anger. First, when he was five years old, Tom killed the family dog.

> That's the one that taught me that I needed to learn to control my temper. Cause I got angry and killed the dog. I don't remember what [my parents] said. Apparently, it was more traumatic for me to kill the dog than it was for whatever they did. I don't remember that part of it. I remember killing the dog.

Then, at age 10, "my brother did something stupid, and I picked him up and put him against the wall with my hands, so I was losing my temper a lot." This continued until Tom was in his late teens, at which time he realized that he was on a dangerous path.

> I started looking back at my life and going through things and figuring out that if I kept going down that route, I was going to end up dead or in prison. So I did a lot of changes to who I was and decided that that was not a route I wanted to go.

This desire to avoid anger and violence bleeds over into his BDSM play. Tom engages in various types of play, though he described a typical scene as involving simply bondage. He described that a scene is "like a meditation, the deeper into it I get, the more focused I get, the more everything drops away." He stated that he feels "calm" during this process. However, he is careful to avoid any type of negative reaction from the submissive.

> I don't like seeing fear or pain. I think it reminds me of the dark side of the personality, and I don't want to be dark, and so I avoid

> the dark side of stuff. I mean, I realize I've got a dark aspect to
> my personality, I just don't want to feed it

Given this, Tom nearly had his worst fear realized when, during breath play, the submissive had an unexpected response and stopped breathing. "It freaked me out because you stop from the breath play, and it takes you a few seconds to notice they're not breathing. And then you're sitting there going "Oh, shit." But luckily I rolled right into doing [CPR].

He was able to revive her after 10 to 20 seconds. However, that effectively ended the scene and their relationship also faltered shortly thereafter. He acknowledged that it was incredibly scary for him, though focuses on the positive aspect of being able to revive her.

Tom's realization of his own "dark side" has shaped his views on sadism and masochism, as well as his opinion of those who practice S&M within the community. He expressed the belief that both are "not healthy," ascribing to the Gorian belief that "sadism is a disease and that for somebody to beat another person for pleasure is a sign of sickness." Tom described being at community events, seeing sadists and masochists play together, and finding it difficult to watch. In the case of a masochist accepting pain as a form of service to her Dominant, Tom says:

> It's torture. It's not – it's not play, it's – it's actually deliberately inflicting pain on somebody that you know they're not going to enjoy. It's actual sadism, and that's not anything I'm remotely into. I kind of view sadists as, like, addicts. They're like an alcohol addict, and you can't really trust an addict because you don't know that somewhere down the line, they might lose control.

This appears to be a projection of Tom's own fear of losing control over his own anger, as he did when he was younger. He dislikes in sadists that which he knows is a part of himself and feels unable to trust. Regardless of the agreement of consent between two other people, he is unable to disassociate the concepts of infliction and reception of pain from forced aggression. For him, they are the same. There is also the possibility that Tom may feel envious of their ability to express aggression while feeling in control of it and having the ability to indulge their sadism. He is self-aware enough that he has recognized his own propensity for violence, and he may realize that should he participate in even consensual sadomasochism, like the alcoholic he references, he would not be able to be trusted. Therefore, he limits his play to areas that cause him minimal anxiety and allow him to feel the most in control.

Dominance as restitution and identification.
Through dominance, Tom is able to contain not only his own primitive aggressive impulses but also that of his partner, which holds a restitutive quality for him. He saw his parents argue, with his mother having the more extreme temper, frequently starting arguments. He may have wondered, on either a conscious or unconscious level, why his father allowed this to continue. However, this is expressed as the statement: "Realistically, nowadays, if they believed in divorce, they would have gotten a divorce."

He recalled his grandparents' marriage, where his grandfather was the dominant force. His perception was that they personified a traditional marriage with pre-postmodern gender roles.

> You go back to the 1950s household, and you look at the advertising from that time period, and there was advertising that existed in magazines and newspapers with the man and the woman over – spanking his wife. That was accepted behavior then. It was only after that that things shifted, and my grandparents are from that time period. So, that was acceptable behavior to them.

He seems to admire both the control that his grandfather exhibited within the home, as well as the implied notion that his grandmother agreed with this, though he stopped short of saying that he ever witnessed his grandfather's control going to the extent of spanking his grandmother ("Well, I don't know. I mean, it never came out, as far as that stuff.") However, the fact that she introduced him to the Gor stories, by giving him the first book in the series, likely played a part in his perception that she endorsed the ways in which the gender roles in the household were divided.

Perhaps he also had the unconscious fantasy that his father would take control of his mother in this way, physically rebuking her tantrums, punishing her anger, and, in the process, making him feel less vulnerable. He also made reference at one point to "women stressing out over issues that they really shouldn't be stressing out over." It is possible that he also wondered why his father allowed her to return to work, concerning herself with an area – finances – that he sees as part of male responsibility. This also speaks to Tom possibly seeing her return to work as a failure on his father's part for not providing financially to the extent that it was not necessary. Finding such fault with both parents, Tom turned to idealizing his grandparents and their marriage, as well as identifying with his grandfather. If he is a dominant force in the relationship, as his grandfather was, then he can escape the perceived difficulties his father had with his mother, possibly allowing for a restitutive relational experience.

Tom also had other disappointments from his parents. From his mother, most notably, were the birth of his younger brother when he was five and her decision to return to work when he was ten. Undesirable change, particularly where the central female object in his life is perceived to be taken away, may have felt intolerable and overwhelming to him at such young ages. His father's frequent changes in employment led to a chaotic and unstable environment for Tom with multiple moves to new houses and schools within a short period of time. Particularly during this time, his grandparents may have functioned as objects of stability and order amongst the chaos. His participation in the Gor sect of BDSM may be his attempt to restitutively recapture the stability that they represented, as well as continue this identification with his grandfather.

Gor: Power exchange and repetition.
Tom was clear that the way in which he practices BDSM is not necessarily about the scene, per se, but rather about the power exchange that occurs between him and his partner, with scenes interspersed at various time intervals and occupying a lower position of priority. "They're kind of a secondary thing to me, they're not really – they're not my primary focus. I can do without play if I have to. It's not an integral part of relationships to me."

Having the hierarchy in place, in which his partner is submissive to him, is what matters most. However, during his adult life, it has been difficult for him to sustain this throughout the length of a relationship. After a certain period of time, the submissive disengages from the power exchange, no longer voluntarily surrendering to him. Despite his efforts, she refuses to reengage, leading to the collapse of the relationship. This appears to be a repeating relational pattern for him. "It's just a matter of as the relationship evolves, sometimes it evolves close together, sometimes it evolves further apart, and sometimes it evolves far enough apart that it just doesn't work anymore."

Additionally, Tom has, in the past, been attracted to women who were chaotic and unstable. He calls them "strong." However, this seems to contradict what he describes as desirable: a traditional relationship that, ultimately, reminds him of his grandparents' marriage. This implies a need for a submissive woman committed to that type of lifestyle as well. It appears highly unlikely that the women he is drawn to will be able to fulfill these needs. His grandmother experienced marriage, motherhood, and femininity as being "1950s" because this was normal and natural for her during that time period. Women today would have to fight against modern convention and their own socialization, as well as pragmatic issues, such as finances, in order to join with Tom in the type of relationship he seeks.

Dominance as a defense against helplessness.
Throughout the interview process, Tom expressed fear of being controlled or trapped. He described this beginning at a young age when his parents and teachers tried to force him to do schoolwork and were unable to. This continued into adulthood with Tom being unwilling to compromise personal values at a job. Even when Tom discussed his sexual identity as a Dominant, he parallelled this to the conflict of freedom versus enslavement.

The desire to remain free of external control also weighs heavily in the fact that he has never been married. He has no desire to get married, which is in direct contradiction to society's ideal of a "traditional" relationship, as is his definition of marriage.

> Marriage doesn't fit my view of what marriage should be. I mean, if marriage was allowed to be what marriage used to be, I might be more inclined to do it. Marriage should allow for [polygamous] relationships, and it doesn't. The government getting involved in marriage has messed a lot of stuff up.

For Tom, the law forbidding polygamy is a type of governmental control to which he is determined not to submit. If he marries, then he will be legally obligated to only one relationship, a construct with which he disagrees. Therefore, he would likely experience marriage in a negative way and has effectively eliminated it as a possibility.

However, there is another, deeper reason for his stance. "I've seen so many marriages go to pot – that they get married, and then things changed and they're stuck in it, and it's so hard to get back out of it." It is likely that he is speaking not only of friends and family members but also his parents' marriage. He witnessed many arguments, no "passionate love" between them, and now a permanent separation because they do not feel able to divorce and be free of each other. There is a fear that he, too, will be trapped and helpless in marriage, as he has seen his parents. Particularly considering the types of relationships Tom has had, his fear may be specific not only to feeling helpless to marriage as an institution but feeling controlled by his partner.

The women that he often chooses, who are "strong," frequently end up with much of the power in the relationship, leaving Tom in a masochistic position. Examples of this include the former girlfriend who, in one instance, threatened suicide and in another, informed his family of his sexual identity. In both cases, each woman sadistically utilized the power that she had in the relationship, with Tom being masochistically helpless. Should he make the decision to marry one of these women, then he may fear reenacting the type of marriage his parents had instead of the more restitutive marriage he witnessed from his grandparents.

Given this, it is possible that Tom constructs these relationships to fail as a protection against marriage. If he chooses a partner who is "strong," then, as mentioned previously, she is unlikely to continue to engage in the power exchange, thus not meeting his stated primary need. If she is not meeting his needs, then he is able to keep the danger that marriage represents at a distance, even though he ultimately sacrifices his happiness. Even if the relationship went well, then he has the moral objection of governmental interference to protect himself from that which he truly perceives as dangerous: marriage itself.

INTERVIEW REACTIONS.

When I first met Tom, I was a bit intimidated by him due to his physical appearance. He is much taller than me and simply has a presence about him that commands attention. Frankly, I associated to Charles Manson, based solely on his physical features, which did nothing to ease my feelings of intimidation and anxiety. However, this soon changed as I witnessed him caring for his infant son. As we continued through the interview process, I came to see him as quite vulnerable and even slightly lost. It felt like he worked very hard to keep people at a distance, and I think the interviews became increasingly difficult for him, the further we went and the more intrusive the questions became. Though he never said so, I sensed that the coexistence of the interviews with his relationship being in flux was at the heart of this. I asked questions that brought to the surface the possibility that this relationship, too, may not last.

There were several interactions with Tom that I felt were significant. During our first interview, he brought up the fact that he recalled some traumatic events from childhood. I paused, saying nothing, because I felt uncertain about whether to go down this path. His use of the word "traumatic" elicited IRB-specific caution within me. During that pause, a great deal happened. First, the pause lasted for seven seconds. There was the audible tick of a clock in the recording, which seemed to emphasize the enormity of those seven seconds. Second, he and I locked eyes. I had my eyebrows raised, nervous, with my mind set that he was free to offer this information, but I was not going to ask for it. Tom, however, was smiling and seemed excited. He seemed to want me to ask, to want to tell me. Seven seconds was how long it took him to decide that he would offer the information.

In our third interview, Tom told me about his former partner who stopped breathing during breath play. I was shocked, stunned, and horrified. My mind struggled to comprehend the possible implications from that type of incident. Yet, I could not stop laughing. As we talked about it on and off the record, I was unable to stop laughing. Even now, when I read that part of the transcript, listen to that part of the interview, or think of that story, I inexplicably begin to laugh. It is the precise opposite of what I feel, and yet I continue to have this reaction. Tom was never really able to talk about his emotions that were tied to that scene – only his relief at having been able to revive her. I am led to wonder if my reaction was, and continues to be, a reflection of his inner thoughts about it. The darker side of his personality finding such an incident amusing, though he would find this much too anxiety-provoking and overwhelming to acknowledge.

Finally, when we needed privacy for our fourth interview, Tom suggested that we simply go into the basement where he and his partner have their play space set up. Though I initially felt a sense of unease about this, I soon saw that this was just like any other interview and the surroundings made no discernible difference. At the end of the interview, during which he discussed the deterioration of his current relationship, I asked him to say a bit about our surroundings. As he talked about the various pieces of equipment, Tom transformed. He seemed alive, content, happy, and at peace, whereas five minutes earlier, he had seemed depressed due to his relational circumstances. He finally seemed to be in his element.

PARTICIPANT 5: ED

Ed is a 44-year-old, Caucasian married male. He lives with his African-American wife of four years in a rural area of North Carolina. He works in the communications field and has been with the same company for several years. Ed is moderately active in the BDSM community, both online and in person, attending events whenever his schedule allows. He is tall, slightly overweight, and balding.

Of note, Ed was the only participant who was concerned about his privacy and wanted to ensure that identifying details would be concealed. He was open and forthcoming during the interview process, speaking in a thoughtful manner with all of his answers. He seemed equally as curious about some questions as the researcher, and the process often felt like a joint search for answers.

Family history.
Ed was born and raised in the same town in which he currently lives. In fact, the house in which he lives with his wife is a family home that has been passed down to him. His parents married late in life, and Ed

was born soon into their marriage. His father was a farmer, and his mother was a homemaker.

Ed's parents had a traditional marriage for the time. "It was a male-led household." His father provided financial support and gave his mother a certain amount of money each month for bills, groceries, and other household needs. He was also the main decision-maker. "If Dad didn't want to do something, it didn't happen." He also explained that they were affectionate "to a lesser degree."

> I think they would kiss every once in a while. I didn't see him in the morning because he was off before I [got up], but I got the impression that they would kiss in the morning. And they would hug every once in a while. Nothing more than that.

When describing the relationship between his parents, Ed said that "it was somewhat dysfunctional, looking at it later." He acknowledged that his father worked a great deal and that his mother expressed frustration with this, wishing that he would spend more time with the family. He said that this means that he does not feel he had an adequate opportunity to observe their relationship in action. However, he presumes that, overall, it was "decent."

When Ed was 16, his father died. He said that other than momentary disbelief, he had, and continues to have, an emotionally blunted reaction.

> I did say, "No, you're kidding," and then after that it was like, "Okay, well, now what?" I miss my father, but I don't have the emotional response that a lot of people have. And my father's passing did affect me, but it's more about missing things that we could have done together, like him showing me how to shave, or telling me what eau du toilette is.

Exacerbating his response is the fact that he is not entirely sure of the cause of his father's death. His father died while plowing a field and was run over by the plow. Therefore, there was uncertainty if he died from his injuries or if he perhaps had a cardiac event that led to secondary injuries from the machinery.

He called his father a "good father," though it seemed apparent throughout the interviews that he wished he had had more time with him. Though his mother was largely the disciplinarian, his father would occasionally step in to assist, which meant that a belt would be used. He estimated that his happened approximately three times.

Ed appeared more ambivalent about his relationship with his mother. After his father's death, it was only the two of them, as Ed is an only child. As he came into adulthood, their relationship became stressed, and he described that she began expressing anger toward him.

> I think she was not happy with my father leaving her. I think she was unhappy with some of my behaviors, that I wasn't being, you know, typical, you know, dating a lot of girls, or that sort of thing. And I wouldn't do what she wanted me to do; I did what I wanted to do.

She resides with family members nearby, requiring full-time care for health issues. Ed has power of attorney and visits her one to two times per month. While he is not responsible for her hands-on care, it was apparent that Ed feels responsible for her well-being and overall quality of life.

When Ed was growing up, sex was not a topic that was ever discussed. Instead of having a discussion with him about sex, his mother bought a series of books about the subject and gave those to him to read. His father was in the military before marriage, and he stated that he had heard from others that his father would make sexual comments and jokes. However, he stated about his mother's younger years: "I think she was a bit of a prude."

Significant relationships.

During the majority of his adult life, Ed has only dated African-American women. He understands this internally as follows:

When I asked white girls out, they would say no and black girls would say yes. After a while, I just sort of stuck with the black girls. And after a while, it got to be where white girls weren't even on the radar. You get reinforced with what's successful, I think.

His relationships with women have historically been short in duration, lasting a matter of months. Largely, these relationships, all rooted in BDSM, began online, and he would later meet the person. Such was the case with Ed and his wife, who is originally from Rhode Island. Ed has been married for four years, in what is his only marriage. They live together with her child from a previous marriage. Ed has no biological children.

There has always been a BDSM component to their relationship. Ed and his wife engage in a Master/slave dynamic, meaning that theirs is a 24/7 power exchange. Ed views this as being service-oriented. She does things in service to him, to please him, and to make his life easier, while he takes care of her.

However, during the interview process, their relationship went through an unexpected transition. His wife requested that her collar, a symbol of commitment to the Master/slave dynamic, be removed. This left Ed shaken and confused. At the conclusion of the interviews, he requested a referral for marriage counseling.

BDSM history.
Ed stated that his family has told stories of him tying up a cousin when he was approximately five years old. He has no memory of this but appears amused by it. As he got older, he described "reading some seriously fucked up porn. The stuff with the girls, you know, and the guys having sex really didn't do anything for me. It was really the more torturing, you know, blood-curdling, dehumanization, objectification-type stuff."

In his mid-twenties, he discovered BDSM forums on the internet and thought "That's why I'm like that." He stated that he neither experienced guilt nor tried to deny his sexual identity, instead embracing it.

When the Master/slave dynamic was in place, Ed's marriage relied upon power exchange. When asked his definition of this, he replied:

> Power exchange is when you can get someone to do something they don't want to do. Without coercion, without force, without saying "Do this or I'll, you know, or I'll do that." It's when you say "Do this because it pleases me. Take this needle and shove it through your skin. Shove it through your nipple. That's a good girl." That's power. The exchange is what she gets – the giving up control to me for her to be able to do that, so it's a two-way street. I can't remember who originally said this, but they said "A Master/slave relationship is an unequal relationship between equals," and I have to agree with that.

Ed identified his main kink as caning, though noted electricity as a close second.

CATEGORIES OF MEANING.

Control as restitution.
Ed explained that the feeling of being out of control is intolerable for him:

> I don't like to drink a lot and don't like to have other people drive my car or drive a car with me in it. I prefer to be the one driving. I hate roller coasters with a passion. I think it all has to do with the fact that I want to be in control of myself and my actions.

Many times during Ed's life, he has experienced being helpless: being bullied in school by classmates who called him a "geek" and a "nerd;" rejection by the girls he found attractive while being pursued by undesirable girls, which increased the bullying behavior; his father's death; and even now, he feels responsible for his mother's care, yet does not seem to want this obligation and is forced to witness her irreversible health decline. Being able to control one aspect of his life completely – women – seems reassuring to Ed and likely serves a restitutive function.

> There's lots of emotions that go through my head. Joy that I have somebody that can take this for me. Pride because she's doing this. Little proud of my skill, too, I'll be honest. There is the whole control aspect, which I don't know if you label control an emotion, but I certainly do.

For Ed, feeling control brings forth many positive emotions to the extent that he experiences control itself as an emotion. He sees this woman whom he loves submitting to him and accepting pain for him, and he feels validated by this. As someone who has experienced rejection by those women considered desirable, this gives him a feeling of power and perhaps superiority. This even extends beyond his marriage to other women who call him "sir" in passing "even if she doesn't realize what that does for me."

> It's not in every situation. But like if I'm being waited on by a waitress or something, or I'm at a strip club and the girl calls me sir, then that gets my dick hard. That's really cool. My mind associates it with control. I'm the one in charge, I'm the one calling the shot, and I like that feeling of being in control and that sense of power.

During a scene, this means that the submissive must not behave in a way that will disrupt the restitution that occurs from Ed being able to feel that power and control. If her behavior in any way is reminiscent of a previous injury he has suffered, then the purpose of the scene evaporates, he again feels helpless, and he abandons the scene.

> I want to be treated with respect. I have no problem with people that want resistance in their scenes. I don't. I don't want you to fight me. I want you to take it. If you're fighting me, it's not service. And I'm big on this whole "pain as a service to me," whole control aspect. If you're taunting me, I'm not in control.

Ed also addressed the question of whether he considers himself to be a sadist. This was a standard question for participants, though it was one with which he struggled to answer in a conventional manner.

That's an interesting question. I enjoy pain, but I don't enjoy pain for pain's sake. I used to think I did. I enjoy pain for the control it gives me over the person. And I don't like playing with masochists because they're into the pain too much. I enjoy the pain because humans don't like suffering, so if I can make someone suffer for me, that is the greatest level of control fulfillment that I know. Is that the classic definition of a sadist? No. Is it sadistic as fuck? Yes. So, I'll let you answer that.

The control he feels by seeing both submission and the acceptance of pain seem to make Ed feel as though he is worthwhile and special. A woman is willing to do these things for him and go through this for him. It invalidates the verbal negativity of his past while simultaneously validating his masculinity and sexuality, which may have been maligned by his mother, who was likely uncomfortable with this when Ed displayed the normal curiosity of a child. All of this is at the core of the restitutive function for him.

However, the dynamics have now changed. His wife made the decision to disengage from their power exchange, taking away that aspect of his power and control. It brings forth the important questions of how will their marriage function now and how will he function in that type of marital dynamic? Will he again feel helpless? Ed and his mother had many power struggles over the years, and one must wonder if he once again feels castrated, though by his wife.

BDSM provides structure.
Ed acknowledged feeling unsure around women, not knowing where boundaries lie, and what is considered acceptable behavior. These types of social graces have always confounded him. Erring on the side of caution, he chose not to approach women in public when he was single, fearing he would offend the person. This is one of the aspects which he most enjoys about BDSM: the structure it provides.

> I need the structure of BDSM. It helps me figure out my relation-
> ships better, gives me a context rather than the free-form rela-
> tionship that seems to be more prevalent in our society. I don't do
> well when I don't have boundaries. I do better when I have a set
> of walls to work within. I need to know what's expected, what I
> can and cannot do and what I should be doing.

BDSM gives him a set of guidelines by which to operate, and he is able
to feel relatively confident that he will be able to both meet his partner's
expectations and have his own expectations met.

However, once his wife's collar was removed, so were the guidelines
for their relationship by which he was used to working. Ed was left
feeling unsure about how this changed the structure of their marriage,
as well as where his boundaries were now repositioned.

> I don't have any experience with vanilla relationships whatsoever.
> It's always about consent, it's always about power exchange, that
> sort of thing. And, for me, when she removed her collar, that to
> me signaled that the relationship was over...But that isn't what
> it meant to her, so that took me a few days to get a hold of and
> grasp. I also have to deal with this whole "Well, if I'm not your
> Master," you know, this was a no safe words, I get to do whatever
> the fuck I want to type of relationship. She's "Well, when can
> we have sex again?" last night, and I'm like "Well, you initiate
> it; you tell me when."

Ed's confusion and vulnerability are evident here. His fear of losing
her takes over and places him in a passive position where he relinquishes
his control to her. Without her collar, he feels she no longer consents
to anything. It removes the entire structure of their marriage for him,
and in many ways, it exposes his inexperience with and immaturity
in relationships. The substitute structure becomes a reverse power
arrangement. He surrenders to her in an effort to avoid what he fears
could be a fatal mistake for their marriage.

Race play.

Though it is not the only type of play in which he engages, Ed enjoys race play, which he described as "role playing racism." "It varies a little bit from person to person, but it usually involves racial epithets." Ed has participated in these types of scenes with different partners over the years, as well as with his wife.

> When we got together, it wasn't about race play. She knew that I did it, but she didn't want to have anything to do with it. We tried it once, she told me to stop. Three months later, she asked me to do it some more. So, she has issues with it, but it is a turn on to a certain degree, but it also causes a lot of anger and rage. It's not safe for me to use those words, but it's fun.

Ed elaborated on the types of language that is used during these scenes. "It's mostly the 'N' word and a few others, you know, 'Tell me,' you know, 'Tell me that you're my N word,' and that sort of a thing."

Due to the nature of these scenes, Ed refrains from engaging in race play in public venues unless it is carried out in a discreet manner.

> I don't do that where other people can tell. Because it is disrespectful to them. It is bringing them into my scene. Just because somebody's Caucasian doesn't mean that they enjoy hearing those words, and I never assume that. It's kind of like bringing other people into the scene. I wouldn't want to hit somebody with my whip with a backstroke. I wouldn't want to hit somebody with my words either that I wasn't intending.

Ed realized that race play has a shocking effect on people, even within the BDSM community. However, he compared this type of roleplay to a Dominant utilizing gender-based verbal humiliation in the scene, questioning the difference, and hinting at hypocrisy. "We never have people say 'Well, you call your wife a dumb cunt; doesn't that affect your view on women?' Well, I don't hear that, but I hear that about race in the scenes." He believed this is because more people are aroused by the verbal humiliation of women, and will acknowledge that, than by race play.

Ed was not concerned that this type of play would damage his relationship. He expected that his wife would talk to him and communicate any concerns that arose, which led him to state his own beliefs.

> I mean, one of the reason why we've been able to engage in race play is because she knows how I feel about her and that it's – that I don't have – I won't say I don't have any negative prejudices against African-Americans because I'm a white guy born and raised in the South. There's probably stuff that I don't realize that I do, and in fact, I know there is. But that's the way it is with everybody. Black people have negative preconceptions about white folks. The thing is to not let them effect how you treat the people. You don't treat a group of people like a group of people. You don't make general assumptions about a group of people based on stereotypes.

Even though Ed acknowledged here that his southern upbringing has influenced his view of African-Americans in some way, he immediately defended against this with the belief that "they do it, too." He seemed to move quickly to a place of comfort, his usual position where he stands strong against the institution of racial discrimination. His brief acknowledgement of negativity in his background appeared to elicit enough anxiety that he felt the need to be seen in a positive light. He continued:

> One of the things I say is, I can never say that I'm not a racist. I have to let the other people decide for themselves whether or not I'm a racist. I can say it all day, every day, but racists do that all the time.

Ed made a concentrated effort to separate himself from those he considers to be racist, and he asserted that if he felt that his view of African-American people was being affected by his BDSM activities, then he would discontinue his participation in race play.

He has played with one partner who was uncomfortable with the terms "Master" and "slave." "I understood. I mean, black woman, white guy." They had a discussion to ensure that both understood expectations and proceeded with the scene. He said he had no problems with this and seemed indifferent to the memory of not being called "Master." The honorific used instead was "Lord."

Interview reactions.

When Ed first contacted me about participating in this study, I went to his online profile to find out more about him, which is what I did for all who expressed interest in this study. As I realized that his relationship dynamic was one of a Caucasian Master with an African-American slave, I had a visceral reaction. I was horrified, angry, and disgusted. My immediate gut reaction was the decision not to allow him to participate.

However, I further considered that decision, and began asking myself questions. Why would I *not* allow him to participate? Was their dynamic automatically not consensual, just by virtue of their races? Did I not want to try to understand the meaning of their relationship from his point of view? Had I not fully realized, having grown up and continuing to reside in the South myself, that seeing this exact dynamic was a viable possibility?

I struggled with judgment and a lack of empathy throughout the interview process, though it became easier as I saw him trying to cope with his deteriorating relationship. The breakdown of his M/s dynamic and his resulting vulnerability truly impacted me. In the second interview, when he told me about his marriage problems, I felt his panic and wanted to comfort him. It also gave me relief to see him in this state, though, because I felt some hope that perhaps he had genuine emotions for his wife. The situation further reminded me that she does hold power in their marriage and is not a slave in the historical sense of the word. It had been hard for me to mentally and emotionally separate the idea of her as a BDSM slave and an actual slave, which was both unusual and significant.

I worked especially hard to understand Ed, his relationship and his internal world. At times, I walked away feeling that Ed likely wondered why I kept harping on the racial aspects, but I needed to understand the intricacies of the phenomenon in order to explain it. I did not yet understand it myself, which was frustrating.

Ed seemed to seek a cautious connection with me. At the end of our first and third interviews, Ed walked me to my car. He continued talking about various things, mainly technology. He also appeared protective about my safety due to the distance I was driving.

At the end of the first two interviews, he tried to encourage the interview to continue longer, saying "You're sure you've got no more questions?" and "We can go longer if you need." After I had turned the recorder off at the end of the third interview, he requested that I turn it back on so that he could add information about his high school experience. At the end of the fourth and fifth interviews, he thanked me. I sensed throughout that he did not want me to have a negative opinion of him.

CHAPTER 5

DISCUSSION

This study sought to bring a deeper, more nuanced understanding of both the relationships and the BDSM scenes of heterosexual southern male Dominants. The goal was to try to access and discover the meaning within the internal world of these participants. Each participant had a unique story and, in some cases, very little in common with each other. Their similarity in demographics – having been raised in the rural South, currently identifying as a Dominant, and being over the age of 40 – are the only manifest commonalities that exist between several participants. Each participant had experienced events in childhood that created a need for restitution. This left open the question of what the quality of their relationships would be. However, what became clear was that most participants valued their partners, her opinions, and her well-being. Most desired a deep connection with his partner that, in some cases, extended to the researcher during the interview process. As the participants described past relationships, many sounded notably chaotic and even masochistic on the part of the Dominant. The fact that one participant's relationship plays with the concept of Antebellum-era slavery was a further opportunity for the exploration of a unique and controversial dynamic, though this participant also culminated in a negative case.

The Negative Case

It became apparent during the interview process with Ed that he was different and distinct from the other participants in significant ways. These differences became more pronounced during the cross-case analysis, as Ed's data contrasted with that of the other Dominants. For this reason, Ed will be discussed separately, focusing on the dissimilarities of the data as well as the meanings of these.

First, while objects of authority play a major role in the restitutive function for all Dominants, with Ed there is also the element of repairing narcissistic injury from adolescent rejection. Ed describes consistent rejection by Caucasian girls to whom he was attracted, which prompted turning his attention toward African-American girls. His attraction seemed to be based on the fact that they did not reinjure him with additional rejection. However, there are questions surrounding what other unconscious factors played into this attraction. Why African-American girls? Did he feel a sense of superiority to or power over them? Conversely, does he, in some way, identify with them as "less than," an identification that he may defend against with sadism?

His interest in Caucasian girls was not completely diminished. As he matured and developed an interest in BDSM, he felt that Caucasian girls were for tying up and African-American girls were for dating. These later blended into the interest of practicing BDSM with African-American women. The way in which these interests developed seems to be indicative of the anger that he felt toward Caucasian women for rejecting him. While other participants also reported adolescent rejection or being a "late bloomer," their reactions to this manifested through BDSM as an enjoyment of control or adoration. Ed's enjoyment of physical sadism and racial humiliation bring a dimension to his BDSM activity that is distinctly different from the others. When combined with his familial and cultural background, it must be considered that Ed may be unconsciously motivated by racism, and possibly even misogyny, in his BDSM participation.

With this in mind, the concept of "BDSM play" must be reexamined and the question asked: when is it no longer play (Tolleson, personal communication, December 11, 2013)? Ed is a man raised in the rural South, whose family farm employed African-American workers. At the least, he was implicitly exposed to the concept of racial hierarchy as normal and acceptable. Ed also acknowledged – then immediately defended against the acknowledgement – that he may have residual racist ideas as a result of his upbringing. Yet, he engages in race scenes with African-American women. If he does harbor racist thoughts, feelings, or attitudes, be these conscious or unconscious, then what does that mean for the scene when race play is involved? His is the one case in which being raised in an area where the discourse on race is still fraught with tension, entitlement, and disparity (as well as the denial by many of these ongoing dynamics) may negatively impact his BDSM interactions.

CROSS-CASE FINDINGS

From the data of the five participants, three main themes emerged. The first, restitution, details a process that occurs from before the BDSM scene begins until after it has ended and includes the element of object usage. Second is the sadomasochistic nature of the emotional aspect of the relationships in which the participants tend to engage. Last, the participants seem to have a desire for connection and relatedness in their relationships, which also extended to the interview process. Last is a discussion of the meanings of gender within BDSM scenes. While not all participants showed evidence of each theme, it was felt that these were the most meaningful aspects that emerged from the totality of the data.

RESTITUTION.

> Perverse mechanisms, which are present in everyone (everyone is neurotic, so everyone is perverse), and perversions (which are, perhaps, just blown-up versions of perverse mechanisms) are

restitutive defenses against earlier, at-first unmanageable, pain (Stoller, 1991, p. 48).

All participants evidenced restitution as a meaningful experience in their BDSM relationships. For most, this also crossed over into the scenes they enacted with their partners, while one participant seemed to gain restitutive benefit solely from the relationship. These will be discussed separately. For four of the five participants, restitution appears to evolve as a process as the scene unfolds, and there seem to be four distinct phases: emotional preparation, scene-specific restitution, fear-based guilt, and aftercare and object usage.

Emotional preparation.
The restitution associated with the BDSM scene is conditional to a large extent. None of these four participants were willing to engage in a scene at any cost. Rather, engagement in the scene was dependent on mutual agreement within the relational dyad on which activities were to occur and that those activities must be consensual, safe, and co-constructed within the framework of play. Without an agreement on each of these terms, then the Dominant would be left with an overwhelming feeling of anxiety, as each tenet allows him to enter into the scene feeling emotionally prepared. He has obtained her consent, learned her limits, attended to safety issues, and is secure in the knowledge that this is merely play. As Stoller (1991) states, "The imitation of humiliation is carefully constructed *never* to produce true humiliation" (p. 21). Through this careful construction, he is able to feel assured that no actual harm will come to his partner.

Additionally, there is the safety mechanism of the safeword, ensuring that he does not hold all of the power. While there is a stated desire to *appear* to have absolute power during BDSM encounters, this is part of the playfulness and fantasy that is being enacted. Even in relationships where no safeword was present, the word "stop" ultimately functioned in the same way, creating the shared power dynamic that is a hallmark of BDSM relationships.

All of this serves the important purpose of allowing the participant to separate himself as much as possible from his aggressive internal objects. If he actually harms his partner, is not vigilant about consent, or becomes truly destructive while in the scene, then he will cross an invisible line, activating a negative identification with the object that he experienced as too controlling, unpredictable, or aggressive. Viewing himself as similar to this object would be damaging to the participant. Stoller (1985) notes:

> The trick is to prevent too much insight from arising in either party, for – the mechanisms understood – there would not be excitement, only wisdom (or arousal and unadorned pleasure, or guilt, anxiety, anger, despair, boredom) (p. 61).

Scene-specific restitution.

> "If you domesticate desire, take the hate away from love and the aggression from sex, whence the glow?" (Dimen, 2001, p. 855)

Once the scene commences, the importance of the fact that this is a co-created play space cannot be minimized. Bader (1993) referred to scenes being "playfully discovered" by BDSM participants (p. 297). Winnicott (1971) stated that, "in playing, and perhaps only in playing, the child or adult is free to be creative" (p. 53). He emphasized the importance of play in children, and these concepts can be extrapolated to adults, particularly once it is considered that nearly all of these participants described domineering parents or parental figures during their childhoods.

The space that is created is an opportunity for the participant to safely regress and play creatively with the interlocking concepts of aggression, love, acceptance, and sexuality without fear of reprisal. However, this type of play has special meaning. Just as McDougall (1985) referred to sadomasochism as "theater," Stoller (1991) also stated that "consensual sadomasochism is theater – an amusement park" (p. 17). He asserted that the person takes an experienced trauma and recreates it within the scene, adding "elements of secrecy, mystery, risk, and illusion" to heighten excitement (p. 18).

The goal of the scene is restitution – mastery over childhood dilemmas in which helplessness was experienced. As part of this mastery, during the scene passive is transformed into active (Stoller, 1991). It is a way in which the participants "[seek] a new reparative object relationship in order to free up their derailed development" (Bader, 1993, p. 296). Chodorow (1992) argues that not only heterosexuality, but all sexuality, including "perversions," can be viewed as a compromise formation. With this in mind, all four of the participants in this category described varying situations that could be seen as childhood dilemmas. Falcor's father used physical violence and intimidation at times, while his mother was submissive. Bob's mother was abusive and manipulative, while his father was passive. Mr. R's mother was the primary disciplinarian, with his alcoholic father only stepping in when necessary. Ed's mother was also the primary disciplinarian, though his father's absence was attributable to work instead of alcohol.

These four scenarios, while mostly different, are similar in that they highlight the helplessness and vulnerability of the participant at the hands of a person who played a formative role in their development. There is also the common thread that many of them may have an unconscious disappointment in the parent who played a passive role in the family and did not protect them from the destructive aggression of another family member. Bader (1993) states that "sometimes the determinative infantile strain-trauma is not abuse, humiliation, or extreme threats to core gender identity but parental weakness, emotional absence, rejection, failures in phase- appropriate mirroring, or all of these" (p. 296). Bob's father would be an example of this, as he failed to protect Bob and his siblings from his sadistic, abusive mother.

For all of these men, dominance is restitutive in that it allows them to express their aggression, discover power and control, and explore their own aggression safely. This can help them to realize that they are different from those whom they have feared or have failed them. The scene also allows them to play with and explore their inherent similarities to the very people from whom they strive to be different. For example, Bob hated his mother for her abusive parenting. However, the scene allows him to explore the control and aggression she enjoyed, taking pleasure in it, without the similarity creating too much anxiety. This is the compromise formation to which Chodorow (1992) referred. There is the unconscious wish to be as powerful as his mother was, abusing others for sadistic pleasure, putting them in positions of misery. This is tempered by the conscious desire to rise above his upbringing, be completely different from her, the protective father he never had. The compromise, then, is carefully explored aggression, with willing partners, in scripted scenes that may have the appearance of his unconscious wishes while having the control Bob requires to both feel safe and provide safety.

Fear-based guilt.
All participants denied feelings of guilt for their activities, and one reason for this may be that they are careful not to violate limits. Among the five participants, safewords have been used by their submissive partners only a handful of times. Bob hypothesizes that he does not push his partners hard enough, and there is likely truth in this. None of them want to experience the feelings evoked by and attached to hearing a safeword, which would likely include guilt for perceived wrongdoing and anxiety at being too closely identified with their bad object.

Due to the scene occurring within the context of play, the introduction of guilt during the scene would negatively color and be apt to effectively end the created play space. Guilt at this point in the process would be disruptive. However, it is likely that as the scene is coming to an end, the Dominant begins to feel unconscious guilt for his aggression against the love object, anxiety that he may have destroyed her, and fear that he may lose her (Klein, 1964; Winnicott, 1969).

In the brief moments between the end of the scene and the beginning of aftercare, it is also possible that these participants experience conflict between unconscious guilt about the powerful feelings he is experiencing that result from the scene and anxiety about the idea that he may have destroyed her with his aggression. The conflict and the fear experienced here propel the Dominant into aftercare.

Aftercare and object usage.
Following the scene, four participants regularly engage in aftercare. While this has the appearance of being a time where attention is focused solely on the submissive, it is actually part of the restitutive process for the participant and is healing for him as well. During aftercare, the Dominant attends to the physical and emotional needs of the submissive post-BDSM play. This looks different between participants, ranging from cuddling and protectiveness to discussion of the activities that have just occurred. For most, this takes place immediately following the scene, while Ed respects his wife's wishes for a few moments to regroup on her own before moving into aftercare.

Winnicott (1969) brought forth the idea that being able to destroy the object and then appreciate the object's survival indicates an ability to use the object. He also stated that, "the idea of the use of an object is related to the capacity to play" (Winnicott, 1969, p. 711). The purpose of aftercare for these Dominants is to transition from the aggression of the play into a calmer, more intimate space wherein they are able to nurture the submissive and ensure that she has survived the scene. He is able to see that his aggression did not destroy her and that it has limitations, even if he feared it did not (Winnicott, 1969; Eigen, 1981). More recently, Kernberg (1995) states that "the beloved presents himself or herself simultaneously as a body which can be penetrated and a consciousness which is impenetrable. . . . The contradictory nature of love is that desire aspires to be fulfilled by the destruction of the desired object, and love discovers that this object is indestructible and cannot be substituted" (p. 44).

The Dominant has been able to enact the unconscious fantasy, likely involving a maternal object, and not only did the object survive but restitutive progress was made. In the process of aftercare, the Dominant is able to separate himself from the other parent he experienced as a child as well, the non-aggressive, passive parent whom he may have experienced as disappointing. He is able to fulfill those protective, soothing functions for which he may have wished and, in doing so, achieves a balance of both respectful, controlled aggression and sensitive protector.

Restitution via the relationship.
Tom is the participant who seems to gain restitutive benefit from the relationship itself instead of the actual scenes. His background is rife with instability and disorder, and BDSM functions as an organizer, much in the way that his grandparents did. The scenes take a backseat to the rules, which help create order. Tom was clear that play is not the focus of his relationships and is not necessary for him, which is evidence that it lacks the restitution he seeks. If the scene brought this about for him, he likely would engage in more play activity and view it as a necessity. Instead, it is the relationship itself, the power dynamics within the structure, and the identification with his grandfather which is evoked that combine as restitutive for Tom. Through this identification, he is able to focus on his grandfather as an object, as he seems to have unconscious disappointment in both of his parents.

The success of restitution.
Given that the participants utilize restitution as part of a healing process, the question should be asked: Is it working? Is this something that is helpful for them? This is a difficult question to answer, given that the behavior continues to occur. Does that mean that BDSM is more a function of compulsion than mastery for some participants? While that is possible, it seems that mastery is the more likely goal. Though participants desired a transformation from passive to active regarding their previous experiences, they notably lacked the desire to act out

harmful aggression. Some even feared their aggressive impulses. Instead, these participants evidenced a desire to recreate the experience in a form acceptable to them, which means repeatedly playing with the concept of aggression instead of acting out actual aggression. Their goal appears to be relief from experienced helplessness.

The question of whether or not this attempt to heal is working for them is difficult to answer, as each participant's situation is unique and dynamic. The definition of success in this instance also depends on the individual. For example, Bob is able to understand and articulate the meaning of his participation in BDSM. He seems to understand the significance of his involvement in particular BDSM activities, such as emotional sadism. Yet, he is mindful of limits and safety issues. He is also able to express anger toward his mother for her abuse and distance himself from her. Given his insight and understanding of the meaning of his activities, as well as his ability to no longer feel helpless regarding his mother, does this constitute success? It is a difficult, if not impossible, standard to determine. However, it is important to note that repetition is a feature that is present is each person's sexuality, whether that includes BDSM, heterosexuality, homosexuality, or any other type of sexual behavior.

SADOMASOCHISM IN OBJECT CHOICE.

The object choice of all five participants was an expected theme (Freud, 1905; Klein, 1964) that clearly emerged. Though it was not specifically listed as a category of meaning, it was discussed at length for each participant in his history, carrying its own weight and significance. Specifically, four of the five participants experienced at least one maternal object from childhood – a mother, grandmother, or both – as a driving, intimidating force.

All but one participant has been married. Of the four who have been married, only one has not been divorced, though his marriage underwent a foundational, structural crisis during the interview process. In all of the marriages/relationships described by the participants, there have been elements of emotional sadism, the withholding of affection and intimacy, or both by the female partners. For example, Falcor felt that his ex-wife was sexually, and later emotionally, withdrawn for much of their marriage, leaving him feeling helpless. All of the men have been placed in an emotionally masochistic position in relationships at some point.

Though they are able to gain control in the bedroom, or for a longer period in some cases, it is clear that these participants are drawn to women who will balance out their need for dominance. Their current partners seem to have stronger personalities and are more dominant themselves in their day-to-day lives. This extends to the relationship, in various ways. For example, one participant needed to check with his submissive before scheduling subsequent interviews to ensure the dates and times worked for her.

All of the participants that I observed interacting with their submissives were affectionate, polite, and nearly deferential toward them, while the submissives I met all seemed to have energetic, "alpha" personalities. Their respective dynamics gave the impression that these women were in charge of the relationships, while the men had a supportive role in the daily operations. One may expect the inverse to be true but that would fail the balance test, leaving each partner feeling either too much in control or with too little power.

Benjamin (1990) discussed the important role of balance in the development of mutual recognition in relationships, beginning with the mother and child.

> The mother has to be able both to set clear boundaries for her child and to recognize the child's will, to both insist on her own independence and respect that of the child—in short, to balance assertion and recognition. If mother and child fail to work out this balance together, omnipotence continues, attributed either to the mother or the self; in neither case can we say that the development

of mutual recognition has been furthered. From the standpoint of intersubjective theory, the ideal resolution of the paradox of recognition is for it to continue as a constant tension between recognizing the other and asserting the self (p. 40).

When BDSM participants engage this tension by alternating the dominant position in the relationship, then the ensuing balance helps them achieve Benjamin's (1990) idea of recognition. Falcor talked at length about the necessity of equality and partnership within the relationship. As demonstrated by many of the past relationships discussed by the participants, when the power dynamic becomes dominated by one person, then neither balance nor recognition is achieved, and the relationship suffers. For example, Tom talked about a former submissive who had become too dependent on him after their relationship had ended. She had medical issues, and what began as him agreeing to help her turned into full-time, long-term dependency that lasted for two years. The result was not only an unbalanced situation but also an unhealthy one. Tom's needs, such as recovering from this relationship ending and potentially making himself available for a new relationship, were not made an equal priority as he masochistically continued to care for her. Though she was dependent on him, she ultimately controlled the relationship with her disability. Recognition in a situation defined by such dependency was impossible.

This required balance and the need for recognition may also explain why most of the participants felt that attempting to construct a dynamic in which they were always in control (or "24/7") was not a realistic option. Two participants had attempted to have this type of structure in place. In Tom's relationship, the continuous power exchange had been negated by the couple's new child and the adjustment that this brought, lending validity to the idea that it is unrealistic for one person to always be in control. Ed also attempted to have a 24/7 power exchange in his marriage. However, his wife disengaged from their power agreement. While this does not automatically bring about a situation where mutual recognition is possible due to other circumstances (see "The Negative

Case"), it does somewhat reverse the dynamics. However, that continues to leave the relationship unbalanced.

THE DESIRE FOR CONNECTION.

Mitchell (1988) states that "the central dynamic struggle throughout life is between the powerful need to establish, maintain, and protect intimate bonds with others and various efforts to escape the pains and dangers of those bonds, the sense of vulnerability, the threat of disappointment, engulfment, exploitation, and loss." This was a struggle that I sensed from the participants, as I felt most of them work to form a connection with me, while a few protected themselves with distance.

Whether by physical contact in the scene or by way of bonding during aftercare, overt relatedness was a priority for participants with regard to their partners. Falcor, Mr. R and Bob described feeling a sense of emotional closeness, connection, or of "being one" with their partner, during or after the BDSM scene. In his discussion of sexual passion, Kernberg (1995) addresses this emotional experience:

> There is an intrinsic contradiction in the combination of these two crucial features of sexual love: the firm boundaries of the self and the constant awareness of the indissoluble separateness of individuals, on the one hand, and the sense of transcendence, of becoming one with the loved person, on the other. The separateness results in loneliness and longing and fear for the frailty of all relations; transcendence in the couple's union brings about the sense of oneness with the world, of permanence and new creation. Loneliness, one might say, is a prerequisite for transcendence (pp. 43-44).

Falcor and Ed also seemed to need a connection with me at the end of the interviews, which I sensed seemed to come too soon or feel abrupt to them. They needed me to talk with them briefly about ordinary things, the equivalent of applying emotional salve after the self-exploration in which they had just engaged, bringing a gradual close to the process.

Alternately, they may have needed that time with me to ensure that they had not destroyed me with the information divulged during the interview. This more directly parallels the aftercare process in which they engage with their submissives. In both scenarios, they seemed to need that connective transitional space between the end of the interview and my departure in order to regroup.

Bob seemed to value the idea of connection, though his fear of vulnerability kept him from fully experiencing it. Many of his more recent scenes had been with submissives he had met online, where there is an implied casualness which he may find comforting and protective. Mitchell (1984) points out that "particularly for patients whose past efforts at relatedness have been severely dashed, warmth, nurturance, connection, can be a frightening prospect" (pp. 491-492). I originally posited that Bob did not seem to fully connect with me, particularly given his acknowledged trepidation at inviting a stranger into his home. I imagined that his focus was likely on returning to a feeling of safety rather than on forging a connection with someone of unknown risk. However, after the study had ended a received a couple of emails him that were, essentially, just touching base. His process of bringing a close to his participation, ensuring that he had not destroyed me, was more delayed, cautious, and distanced, which was in keeping with the glimpse I had gotten into his internal world.

Mr. R seemed ambivalent about bonding with me, though he also held this attitude about aftercare in casual scenes. Where connection was clearly important to him was in the context of his relationship. This leads me to conclude that he is more discriminating about with whom he connects on an emotional level. He realizes that his partner is safe, though casual partners, as well as a researcher, are unknown variables. While he is careful to make sure his partners in casual scenes have survived and will continue to survive, he reveals nothing of himself that will result in a reciprocal connection. This is reserved for the sanctity of his committed relationship.

Tom also did not seem to connect on a significant emotional level with me, and he also did not seem to put a great deal of emphasis on aftercare. Given that he was unhappy in his relationship at the time, it may have felt difficult to make himself vulnerable in this way. In his relationship, he may find it difficult to maintain a connection with his partner given the emotional depletion he seemed to be experiencing during the course of the interviews.

In all three cases where the participants kept emotional distance from me, there seems to be the commonality of the BDSM scene providing the opportunity for these men to safely traverse their personal boundaries into an arena where they are able to safely and uniquely experience intimacy (Tolleson, personal communication, November 14, 2013). Bob, for example, maintained that scenes create a bond between the people involved and stated that, "it's not much stronger activity between two people than having sex – unless it's kinky sex." Mr. R described a part of a scene with his submissive.

> So, when I put her cuffs on her, and her collar last night—you know, had her on the floor in front of me, and was petting her, and stroking her, and, you know, we were sharing some intimacy within the confines of our D/s relationship, and then, as I was trying to feed her pizza, the pizza fell all over the place and that turned into a giggle fit. In an idealized vanilla relationship, everybody would have this level of connection and affection, and I just don't believe most people do that, regardless of if there's vanilla or power exchange. I certainly never encountered anything like this in my previous relationships, and she didn't either.

The concepts of connection here seem to relate to Tolpin's (1997) idea that part of the pleasure derived from sex and sexuality is that the Other shares in the experience with us. There is a thrill in the knowledge that we are not alone either in our desires and fantasies or our willingness to act these out, even if it is categorized as a "perversion" (Tolpin, 1997).

With Tom, I was able to observe the transformation of his mood and facial expressions from depressed and withdrawn to engaging and excited as we moved from discussing the state of his relationship to the various pieces of equipment in his home. These scenarios and statements demonstrate either the likely capacity for or actual ability to experience connection, relatedness, and intimacy within the BDSM scene.

GENDER.

Gender has not been directly addressed in these findings. The reason for this is that BDSM is a dynamic that functions based on voluntary playfulness with power. The dyad bends and distorts, redefines, and exchanges the power that exists between them, usually for a predetermined period of time. This occurs within the dyad regardless of the gender(s) of the participants – male Dominant/female submission, female Domme/male submissive, male Dominant/male submissive, female Domme/female submissive, plus the possibility of transgender and polyamorous participant constellations.

The fact that I chose to study male Dominants who are heterosexual, and thus partnered with female submissives, is not a statement about gender-driven power dynamics. Any other gender constellation could have been selected for study, and the BDSM power dynamic between the couple would still be the most important element within the foreground of the scene. Gender is ever-present, but it remains in the background (Shelby, personal communication, January 31, 2014), informing each person's internal dialogue and experience, such as with the participant's efforts at restitution and history of intimidating maternal objects.

Yost (2007) studied a BDSM population that included Dominants, submissives, and switches. She states:

Practitioners with the S/M community have argued that gender is not the most important factor organising S/M sexuality, and the current study supports this claim. Role identity, not gender, largely determined sexual fantasy content and the location of sexual pleasure.

Gemberling et al. (2015) reinforces this with their assertion that power dynamics are the most important factor in BDSM as a sexual orientation.

Other BDSM dyads, such as male dominant/male submissive and female domme/female submissive, function with the same emphasis on the power exchange as a heterosexual couple. Sexual orientation, like gender, also falls into the background. Tom provides a good example of how this happens in a heterosexual person.

> I've done a few scenes where there was no sexual interest. I mean I have spanked big chunky, hairy guys; I've got absolutely zero sexual interest in them. But I'll still do a spanking scene with them. They asked, and I wasn't doing anything, and they enjoyed being spanked. It was a spanking scene. That's all it was. Now they may have gotten some sexual enjoyment out of it. I don't know, you would have to ask them. But for me, there wasn't anything sexual about that.

What is illustrated here is that neither gender nor sexual orientation are determining factors in a scene but rather the ability to engage in a power exchange. If one person is able to surrender to another person, who is able to take control, then the scene can successfully proceed.

When thinking about implications of gender in heterosexual dyads, those who identify as switches must also be considered. A male or female may take on the dominant role in one particular scene, and then change to a submissive role in the next. This demonstrates a certain fluidity within the BDSM regarding role, gender, orientation and identity.

Bader (1993) notes that there is sometimes the implication "that manifest relations of power are the real ones, that the role of woman-as-object is always deeply anchored in the subjective experience of both actors, and that the result is always the negation of women's sexual agency" (p. 297). This is a dangerous assumption, and is possibly one of the fallacies that lead the analytic community to pathologize BDSM activities and, by extension, its community members. "I think that a view of healthy sexuality that a priori excludes any complementaries involving dominance and submission, particularly if they are along traditional gender lines, can carry with it a repressive morality" (Bader, 1993, p. 297).

With the exception of Ed, the power dynamics in these cases were clearly co-constructed. The submissives had largely determined what activities would occur through communication prior to the scene, they had made their limits known, and they had the ability to call a halt to the scene at any given time. Several participants mentioned the fact that submissives truly hold the power in these interactions. Bob stated that a goal of the scene for Dominants is to "serve the sub" and her needs. In other words, the Dominant may hold and wield the flogger, but he flogs for her pleasure. Tom stated that, "in my view, play is a form of service. Doms are in service to their submissives. It's both ways, or it is if it's a healthy relationship anyway."

Again, gender certainly informs some of this, but it is relegated to the background while the power dynamics take center stage during the scene. The fact that a man is in control of a woman for the duration of the scene matters not. What matters is that a Dominant is in control of a submissive for the duration of the scene, as agreed upon and consented to. Their genders are less important than the roles they play to fulfill their individual psychological needs.

IMPLICATIONS FOR THEORY AND PRACTICE

In this study, several concepts emerged that lend themselves to the reexamination of the ways in which we conceptualize sexuality in the literature. In particular, the ideas that the participants were working at restitution, valued a connection with their partners, and, in most cases, were capable of object usage contradicts the notion of their sexual interactions being pathological. In fact, all of these behaviors are what we expect to see in healthy individuals.

Stoller (1991) states that "the name calling inside our explanations hides a professional bias: Analysts dislike and fear perversion" (p. 48). Throughout a great deal of psychoanalytic literature, there is the belief that sexual behavior which deviates from "normative" sexuality is perverse and that perversions are pathological. However, this type of thinking is reductionistic toward a set of complex behaviors that merit view from a psychoholistic perspective. Tolleson (2005) states:

> Psychopathology cannot be assumed from the observation of behavior alone, but can only be gleaned from the analysis of meaning. So, for example, to witness an angry outburst in a person tells us nothing about the relative health or illness of his psyche (to behave in an angry way may represent extreme health or extreme illness, we just don't know from the behavior alone). In the same sense, perversion is not reducible to a specific sexual *behavior*, but must refer to the meaning of that sexual behavior, or the fantasies that inform it (p. 1).

It has only been more recently that thought and consideration have been given to the idea that perhaps the scope of what constitutes a perversion is much narrower than originally thought. Within postmodern thinking, there have been some who have begun to acknowledge that fantasies of domination and submission can fall within the scope of "normative." Davies (2006) states:

> These are the fantasies commonly associated with what I have termed the darker side of Eros, or what we have come to think of as "the perverse," with a small "p." Let me pause here for a moment to elaborate that I am using the controversial term perversion, always in quotations in this paper, to denote a kind of universal, polymorphously powerful, almost always shame-riddled aspect of human sexual imagination, an aspect of sexual fantasy and

behavior that may be experienced as deviant but that, to my own way of thinking and implicit in the thesis of this paper, is anything but. These are the fantasies we think of as "a little dirtier," "a little rougher," and often "a little hotter." These are the fantasies that we all have and about which we are all ashamed to speak "I pray that love may never come to me with murderous intent, / In rhythms measureless and wild." These are the fantasies that involve aggression, shame, domination, and submission, the power dimensions of who loves who more, who needs who more, the will he come, the will she stay, the must I tie her up, him down to hold, arouse, titillate, and drive to distraction and surrender. These are the fantasies that unite the self with a taunting, teasing, ever- alluring, bad exciting object. Indeed one might suggest that an individual's history of playful "perversion" in fact holds his relationship to this exciting and elusive other. In fact we might consider that to not have such fantasies is more pathological than the having of them, as their absence would denote the continued dissociation into adulthood of a system of erotic sexual elaboration that is developmentally inescapable (p. 674).

This represents a humanistic, empathic and necessary shift, recognizing both the individuality of sexual expression and the evolving comfort that is felt with the realization of some aspects of the "dark Eros." However, the challenge may lie in accepting that the concept of "normative" sexual behavior is not only nearly impossible to define in a universal manner but is damaging in many cases. Once you deem a population of people to be "normal," then those excluded from that population are automatically "abnormal," a dangerous implication.

Throughout this study, the concept of consent has repeatedly been broached as a cornerstone, a prerequisite, of sexual interaction. Just as with "normative" sexual activity, consent is required in order to proceed. However, in contrast with that which is "normative," each individual act must gain consent within a BDSM scene, a heightened standard. Additionally, activities and limitations are explicitly discussed and agreed upon in advance between partners. This emphasizes the important role played by communication in the BDSM scene. Stoller (1991) states:

Constant high attention to one's partner's experience is more caring and safer than the blundering, ignorant, noncommunicating obtuseness that governs so many "normal" people's erotic motions. . . . We should distinguish those who harm from those who, in trying to undo the effects of harm inflicted on them early in life, play at harm" (p. 21).

However, the findings of this study broach an interesting dilemma regarding consent. When two people consent to the activities taking place, that consent is valid for the conscious intentions which each have been able to communicate. If one person holds racist or misogynistic views, then they likely will not be capable of acknowledging that to their partner. How, then, is the issue of consent to be addressed regarding unconscious motivations and attitudes, such as with the case of Ed? Even if consent exists in these relationships, when the unconscious attitude negatively affects the partner, is the declaration of consent still valid? This is a question for which I have no answer, though I feel it is an important issue that warrants consideration. However, the only certainty may be that one is never quite capable of obtaining full disclosure of that to which we are consenting.

When engaging in BDSM activities, if the line from "play" to "non-play" is crossed, then this has implications in the realm of gender relations. Does BDSM then become another vehicle for the subjugation of women, at least in a male/female relationship? The BDSM community works to differentiate the activities which occur in a scene from abuse; indeed, most participants stressed the importance of their partner's feelings and experience. However, when the needs, experience, and safety of the submissive partner become less important than the desire to act out a fantasy, regardless of the potential harm to the person and/or relationship, then the line has been crossed. Equality and consent no longer exist, if they ever did, and the situation becomes pathologically perverse, even abusive.

Lichtenberg's (2010) definition of sexual perversion presents several concepts, including consent, as foundational, and this may be the most useful view, from a standpoint of depathologizing activities traditionally considered perverse.

> In a sociological situation in which paired relationships are of loving equals, and each person's subjectivity and desire are recognized and respected by the other, then consensually accepted sexual practices, whether procreative or not, cannot be regarded as perverse in a psychoanalytic "diagnostic" sense. The historic list of sadomasochism, fetishism, mutual masturbation, voyeurism, exhibitionism, cross dressing, and homosexuality when practiced as a consensual choice between two sensitive, caring individuals, constitutes an expression of sexual desire compatible with attachment and romantic love. Playing at power, say in a sadomasochistic script that can shift between which partner has it and which does not, is within lustful love; angrily, violently, vengefully wielding sexual power is lust without love. The key words that differentiate are playful, sensitive, recognizing and respecting the subjectivity and desire of the other, and equality and consensuality of choice – all components, outgrowths, and manifestations of love (p. 8).

The issue of the perversions and psychopathology is a popular debate within the psychoanalytic community. This study demonstrates a distinct comparison between four BDSM participants who are focused on healthy restitution and relatedness with their partners and then one participant who emerges as different. While Ed's case may be unsettling, it affords clinicians the opportunity to see an example of a problematic BDSM relationship and the dynamics that set it apart from the other cases. This provides more concrete evidence for clinicians to utilize as a guide when working with patients from the BDSM community.

Where we are positioned theoretically determines our therapeutic/analytic stance with patients, which can be of critical importance in our work with alternative sexualities. During my interviews with all of the participants, many topics arose that were outside of the scope of the final analysis. One of these issues, raised briefly by multiple participants, is of critical significance to clinicians. The participants have engaged in cathartic play – scenes aimed at providing psychological and emotional relief to the submissive. This is often due to deeper issues, such as trauma. One participant addressed this:

> A: Some of it is okay, if it's minor issues, but anything that's major like traumatic experiences from their childhood and stuff like that, they need stuff deeper than what an untrained Dom is going to be able to give them. I mean, we all have a certain amount of psychological experience from life.
>
> Q: Do you think that that type of play is safe?
>
> A: No. You're deliberately stepping on an emotional landmine, which is potentially going to leave them in an emotional state where they're not capable of dealing with reality.

This is clearly a situation where BDSM-identified people are feeling left to their own devices to try and resolve their suffering. Given that the mental health community has a long history of negatively categorizing those who engage in sexual perversions, it may be possible that members of the BDSM community are declining to seek treatment for fear of being labeled "perverse" or of their sexuality becoming the unnecessary focus of treatment. This is problematic, as it places one or the other partner in a BDSM relationship in the compromised position of "lay therapist" and, even with a cathartic release during a scene, the traumatized individual has only gained temporary relief. It is a near certainty that this type of dynamic will eventually become corrosive to the relationship.

Others are beginning to conceptualize kink as a sexual orientation (Hoff, 2006; Gemberling, et al., 2015), which means that clinicians will likely begin to see more of this population in their practices as its members increasingly become comfortable and feel accepted by society. If other disciplines are beginning to depathologize BDSM/kink to the point that it is being reformulated as a possible sexual orientation, then psychoanalysts must also reconsider their theoretical positions and where they have situated kink in their clinical work. Williams (2015) argues that "social work needs a good spanking" for its failure to welcome new research and scholarship. Certainly, psychoanalysis does not want to remain stuck in outdated beliefs to the point where it joins social work in Williams' assessment. However, as Hoff (2006) pointed out, a great deal of education must be provided to psychotherapists to prevent stigmatization, inadequate or unethical practice, negative client experiences, avoidable countertransference reactions, and mostly importantly, harm to those seeking help.

From a practice perspective, it is critical that mental health practitioners reconsider the theoretical positions that inform our work with those who engage in "perverse" sexuality. By imposing morality instead of maintaining an empathic stance, we have unintentionally denied services to those who need them. In an era where there is growing discussion around increasing access to psychotherapy, creating a non-judgmental, welcoming environment for individuals in our offices, regardless of their sexuality, should be the primary focus.

SUMMARY

There were many similarities amongst the participants when all of their categories of meaning were comparatively analyzed. All participants in this study showed evidence of seeking restitution for childhood experiences through BDSM scenes and activities. However, in the quest to do this, their relationships with women were distinctively chaotic and sometimes masochistic in nature. Most participants seemed to have the desire to connect with his partner on a deep, meaningful, and emotionally intimate level. In some cases, this need for connection extended to the researcher during the interview process.

The negative case showed the differences in the ways that BDSM relationships function and that these differences are not always healthy. It provides a window into the potentially harmful unconscious motivations that this participant may have with his BDSM participation. It also provides a comparison between his relationship and those of the other participants for the reader to gain perspective regarding the issue of psychopathology.

References

BDSM Dictionary. *BDSM Education.* Retrieved February 4, 2010, from http://www.bdsm-education.com/dictionary.html

BDSM Terms and Definitions. *Yes Master: BDSM resource site.* Retrieved from http://www.fire-runner.com/bdsmterms.htm

Bader, M. J. (1993). Adaptive sadomasochism and psychological growth. *Psychoanalytic Dialogues, 3*(2), 279-300.

Bak, R. C. (1974). Distortions of the concept of fetishism. *The Psychoanalytic Study of the Child, 29,* 191-214.

Benjamin, J. (1988). *The bonds of love: Psychoanalysis, feminism, and the problem of domination.* New York: Pantheon Books.

Benjamin, J. (1990). An outline of intersubjectivity: The development of recognition. *Psychoanalytic Psychology, 7S,* 33-46.

Benjamin, J. (1990). Recognition and destruction: An outline of intersubjectivity. *Like subjects, love objects: Essays on recognition and sexual difference.* New Haven: Yale University Press.

Blanchot, M. (1965). *The Marquis de Sade: Justine, philosophy in the bedroom, and other writings* (pp. 37-72). New York: Grove Press.

Blos, P. (1991). Sadomasochism and the defense against recall of painful affect. *Journal of the American Psychoanalytic Association, 39,* 417-455.

Board, S. B. a. C. Urban and rural population in South Carolina. Retrieved July 12, 2011, from http://www.sccommunityprofiles.org/scpages/sc_urban.php?COUNTYID=47

Boles, J. B. (1999). The southern way of religion. *The Virginia Quarterly Review, 75*(2), 226-247.

Bollas, C. (1984). Loving Hate. *Annual of Psychoanalysis, 12,* 221-237.

Bollas, C. (1987). Extractive introjections. *The shadow of the object: Psychoanalysis of the unthought known* (pp. 157-172). New York: Columbia University Press.

Brame, G. (2000). BDSM/Fetish demographics survey.

Burch, B. (1998). Lesbian sexuality/female sexuality searching for sexual subjectivity. *Psychoanalytic Review, 85*(3), 349-372.

Census, B. (1994). *The urban and rural classifications.*

Chodorow, N. (1992). Heterosexuality as a compromise formation: Reflections on the psychoanalytic theory of sexual development. *Psychoanalysis and Contemporary Thought, 15,* 267-304.

Chodorow, N. (2005). Gender on the modern-postmodern and classical-relational divide: Untangling history and epistemology. *Journal of the American Psychoanalytic Association, 53,* 1097-1118.

Clark, L. P. (1927). A tentative formulation of the origin of sadomasochism. *Psychoanalytic Review, 14*(1), 85-88.

Compton, A. (1985). The concept of identification in the work of Freud, Ferenczi, and Abraham: a review and commentary. *Psychoanalytic Quarterly, 54,* 200-234.

Cross, P. A., & Matheson, K. (2006). Understanding sadomasochism: An empirical examination of four perspectives. In P. J. Kleinplatz & C. Moser (Eds.), *Sadomasochism: Powerful pleasures* (pp. 133-166). Binghamton, NY: Harrington Park Press.

Dancer, P. L., Kleinplatz, P. J., & Moser, C. (2006). 24/7 SM slavery. In P. J. Kleinplatz & C. Moser (Eds.), *Sadomasochism: Powerful pleasures* (pp. 81-101). Binghamton, NY: Harrington Park Press.

Davies, J. M. (2006). The times we sizzle, and the times we sigh: The multiple erotics of arousal, anticipation, and release. *Psychoanalytic Dialogues, 16,* 665-686.

dePeyer, J. (2002). Private terrors: Sexualized aggression and a psychoanalyst's fear of her patient. *Psychoanalytic Dialogues, 12*(4), 509-530.

Dimen, M. (1991). Commentary on Michael J. Bader's "Adaptive sado-masochism and psychological growth". *Psychoanalytic Dialogues, 3*, 301-308.

Dimen, M. (2001). Perversion is us?: Eight notes. *Psychoanalytic Dialogues, 11*, 825-860.

Downing, L. (2007). Beyond Safety: Erotic Asphyxiation and the Limits of SM Discourse. In D. Langdridge & M. Barker (Eds.), *Safe, sane and consensual: Contemporary perspectives on sadomasochism* (pp. 119-132). New York: Palgrave Macmillan.

Eigen, M. (1981). The area of faith in Winnicott, Lacan and Bion. *The International Journal of Psychoanalysis, 62*, 413-433.

Ellis, H. (1995). Studies in the psychology of sex. In T. S. Weinberg (Ed.), *S&M: Studies in Dominance and Submission* (pp. 37-40). Amherst, NY: Prometheus.

Fairbairn, W. (1952). The repression and the return of bad objects (with special reference to the 'war neuroses.' *Psychoanalytic Studies of the Personality* (pp. 59-81). London: Rutledge.

Filho, J., Oliveira, L., Sanches, N., Ceccarelli, P., Ferreira, R., Abras, R., & Foscarini, S. (2005). Trauma, perversion and marital bond. *International Forum of Psychoanalysis, 14*(3/4), 153-158.

Flynt, W. (2006). Country churches. In S. S. Hill (Ed.), *The new encyclopedia of southern culture* (Vol. Religion, pp. 49-54). Chapel Hill: The University of North Carolina Press.

Frazier, T. (2006). Women and religion. In S. S. Hill (Ed.), *The new encyclopedia of southern culture* (Vol. 1, pp. 160-164). Chapel Hill, NC: The University of North Carolina Press.

Freud, A. (1936). *The writings of Anna Freud, volume II: The ego and the mechanisms of defense.* Madison, CT: International Universities Press, Inc.

Freud, S. (1905). *The standard edition of the complete psychological works of Sigmund Freud, volume VII (1901-1905): A case of hysteria, three essays on sexuality and other works* (Vol. 7). London: The Hogarth Press and the Institute of Psychoanalysis.

Freud, S. (1915). Instincts and their vicissitudes. *The standard edition of the complete psychological works of Sigmund Freud, volume XIV (1914-1916): On the history of the psycho-analytic movement, papers on metapsychology and other works* (Vol. 14, pp. 109-140). London: The Hogarth Press and the Institute of Psycho-analysis.

Freud, S. (1920). Beyond the pleasure principle. *The standard edition of the complete psychological works of Sigmund Freud, volume XVIII (1920-1922): Beyond the pleasure principle, group psychology and other works.* London: The Hogarth Press and the Institute of Psychoanalysis.

Freud, S. (1920). A child is being beaten: A contribution to the study of the origin of sexual perversions. *International Journal of Psycho-Analysis, 1*, 371-395.

Freud, S. (1921). *Group psychology and the analysis of the ego. The standard edition of the complete psychological works of Sigmund Freud, volume XVIII (1920-1922): Beyond the pleasure principle, group psychology and other works, 65-144.*

Freud, S. (1927). Fetishism. *The standard edition of the complete psychological works of Sigmund Freud, volume XXI (1927-1931): The future of an illusion, civilization and its discontents, and other works, 147-158.*

Freud, S. (1986). Three essays on the theory of sexuality. I: The sexual aberrations. In P. Buckley (Ed.), *Essential papers on object relations* (pp. 5-39). New York: New York University Press.

Gemberling, T., Cramer, R,. & Miller, R. (2015). BDSM as Sexual Orientation: A Comparison to Lesbian, Gay, and Bisexual Sexuality. *Journal of Positive Sexuality, 1*(3), 37-43. Retrieved from http://journalofpositivesexuality.org/wp-content/uploads/2015/11/BDSM-as-Sexual-Orientation-Gemberling-Cramer-Miller.pdf

Ghent, E. (1990). Masochism, submission, surrender—masochism as a perversion of surrender. *Contemporary Psychoanalysis, 26*, 108-136.

Gillespie, W. H. (1956). The general theory of sexual perversion. *International Journal of Psycho-Analysis, 37*, 396-403.

Glasser, M. (1986). Identification and its vicissitudes as observed in the perversions. *International Journal of Psycho-Analysis, 67*, 9-16.

Goldberg, A. (1995). *The problem of perversion*. New Haven: Yale University Press.

Harris, A. (2003). Misogyny: Hatred at close range. H*ating in the first person plural: psychoanalytic essays on racism, homophobia, misogyny and terror* (pp. 249-278). New York: The Other Press.

Hill, S. S. (2006). Religion. In S. S. Hill (Ed.), *The new encyclopedia of southern culture* (Vol. Religion, pp. 1-20). Chapel Hill: The University of North Carolina Press.

Hodges, D. (1961). Normal sadism and immoralism. *Psychoanalytic Review, 48B*(2), 33-40.

Hoff, G. (2006). Power and Love: Sadomasochistic Practices in Long-Term Committed Relationships. Electronic Journal of Human Sexuality, 9. Retrieved from http://www.ejhs.org/volume9/Hoff-abst.htm

Hoffman, L. (2000). Sexuality as compromise formation. *Journal of Clinical Psychoanalysis, 9*, 301-305.

Jukes, A. (1993). Violence, helplessness, vulnerability and male sexuality. *Free Associations, 4*(1), 25-43.

Kaplan, S. (1957). Panel reports - The latency period. *Journal of the American Psychoanalytic Association, 5*, 525-539.

Kernberg, O. (1991). Sadomasochism, sexual excitement, and perversion. *Journal of the American Psychoanalytic Association, 39*, 333-363.

Kernberg, O. (1998). Aggression, hatred, and social violence. *Canadian Journal of Psychoanalysis, 6*(2), 191-206.

Kernberg, O. F. (1992). Chapter 2: The psychopathology of hatred. *Aggression in personality disorders and perversions* (pp. 21-32). New Haven, CT: Yale University Press.

Klein, M. (1935). A contribution to the psychogenesis of manic-depressive states. *International Journal of Psycho-Analysis, 16*, 145-175.

Klein, M. (1952). Some theoretical conclusions regarding the emotional life of the infant. In M. R. Khan (Ed.), *Envy and gratitude and other works 1946–1963*. London: The Hogarth Press and the Institute of Psycho-Analysis.

Klein, M., & Riviere, J. (1964). *Love, hate and reparation*. New York: W.W. Norton & Company, Inc.

Kleinplatz, P. J., & Moser, C. (2007). Is SM pathological? In D. Langdridge & M. Barker (Eds.), *Safe, sane and consensual: Contemporary perspectives on sadomasochism* (pp. 55-62). New York: Palgrave Macmillan.

Kolmes, K., Stock, W., & Moser, C. (2006). Investigating bias in psychotherapy with BDSM clients. In P. Kleinplatz & C. Moser (Eds.), *Sadomasochism: Powerful pleasures* (pp. 301-324). Binghamton, NY: Harrington Park Press.

Kosmin, B., & Mayer, E. (2001). American religious identification survey. New York City: The Graduate Center of the City University of New York.

Krafft-Ebing, R. v. (1892). *Psychopathia sexualis*. Philadelphia: F.A. Davis Company.

Langdridge, D., & Barker, M. (2007). Situating sadomasochism. *Safe, sane and consensual: Contemporary perspectives on sadomasochism* (pp. 3-9). New York: Palgrave Macmillan.

LaPlanche, J., & Pontalis, J. P. (1973). *The language of psychoanalysis: Translated by Donald Nicholson-Smith*. London: The Hogarth Press and the Institute of Psycho-Analysis.

Leonoff, A. (1997). Destruo ergo sum: Towards a psychoanalytic understanding of sadism. *Canadian Journal of Psychoanalysis, 5*(1), 95-112.

Lichtenberg, J. (2010). *Love has a lot to do*. Paper presented at the Symposium 2010: Love, sex & passion, Mount Sinai Medical Center. http://internationalpsychoanalysis.net/wp-content/uploads/2010/03/LichtenbergPaperFinalLoveHastoDo.pdf

Loewenberg, P. (1988). Psychoanalytic models of history: Freud and after. In W. M. Runyan (Ed.), *Psychology and historical interpretation* (pp. 126-165). New York: Oxford University Press.

Lowe, W. (1983). The Playboy readers' sex survey.

McDougall, J. (1986). Identifications, neoneeds and neosexualities. *The International Journal of Psychoanalysis, 67*, 19-30.

McDougall, J. (2000). Sexuality and the neosexual. *Modern Psychoanalysis, 25*(2), 155-167.

Meyer, J. K., & Levin, F. M. (1990). Sadism and masochism in neurosis and symptom formation. *Journal of the American Psychoanalytic Association, 38*, 789-805.

Mitchell, S. (1984). Object relations theories and the development tilt. *Contemporary Psychoanalysis, 204*, 473-499.

Mollinger, R. (1982). Sadomasochism and developmental stages. *Psychoanalytic Review, 69*(3), 379-389.

Moore, T. (1995). *Dark eros: The imagination of sadism.* New York: Spring.

Moser, C., & Kleinplatz, P. J. (2006). Introduction: The state of our knowledge on SM. *Sadomasochism: Powerful pleasures* (pp. 1-16). Binghamton, NY: Harrington Park Press.

Newmahr, S. (2010). Rethinking kink: Sadomasochism as serious leisure. *Qualitative Sociology, 33*(3), DOI: 10.1007/s11133-010-9158-9

Nichols, M. (2006). Psychotherapeutic issues with "kinky" clients: Clinical problems, yours and theirs. In P. J. Kleinplatz & C. Moser (Eds.), *Sadomasochism: Powerful pleasures* (pp. 281-300). Binghamton, NY: Harrington Park Press.

Nordling, N., Sandnabba, N. K., Santtila, P., & Alison, L. (2006). Differences and similarities between gay and straight individuals involved in the sadomasochistic subculture. In P. J. Kleinplatz & C. Moser (Eds.), *Sadomasochism: Powerful pleasures* (pp. 41-57). Binghamton, NY: Harrington Park Press.

Norman, C. E. (2007). Religion and food. In J. T. Edge (Ed.), *The new encyclopedia of southern culture* (Vol. 7: Foodways, pp. 95-100). Chapel Hill, North Carolina: The University of North Carolina Press.

Olsen, C. J. (2009). Paternalism. In N. Bercaw & T. Ownby (Eds.), *The new encyclopedia of southern culture* (Vol. Gender, pp. 201-204). Chapel Hill: The University of North Carolina Press.

Parsons, M. (2000). Sexuality and perversion a hundred years on: Discovering what Freud discovered. *International Journal of Psycho-Analysis, 81*(1), 37-50.

Posner, B., Glickman, R., Taylor, E., Canfield, J., & Cyr, F. (2001). In search of Winnicott's aggression. *The Psychoanalytic Study of the Child, 56,* 171-190.

Prior, E., Williams, D. (2015). Does BDSM Power Exchange Among Women Reflect Casual Leisure? An Exploratory Qualitative Study. *Journal of Positive Sexuality, 1*(1), 12-15. Retrieved from http://journalofpositivesexuality.org/wp-content/uploads/2015/02/Does-BDSM-Power-Exchange-Among-Women-Reflect-Casual-Leisure-Prior-Williams.pdf

Reiersol, O., & Skeid, S. (2006). The ICD diagnoses of fetishism and sadomasochism. In P. J. Kleinplatz & C. Moser (Eds.), *Sadomasochism: Powerful pleasures* (pp. 243-262). Binghamton, NY: Harrington Park Press.

Richards, A. K. (2003). A fresh look at perversion. *Journal of the American Psychoanalytic Association, 51*(4), 1199-1218.

Richter, J., de Visser, R., Rissel, C., Grulich, A., & Smith, A. (2008). Demographic and psychological features of participants in bondage and discipline, "sadomasochism" or dominance and submission (BDSM): Data from a national survey. *Journal of Sexual Medicine, 5,* 1660-1668. doi: 10.111/j.1743-6109.2008.00795.x

Roiphe, H., & Galenson, E. (1987). Preoedipal roots of perversion. *Psychoanalytic Inquiry, 7,* 415-430.

Rothstein, A. (1991). Sadomasochism in the neuroses conceived of as a pathological compromise formation. *Journal of the American Psychoanalytic Association, 39,* 363-402.

Runyan, W. (1988). *Psychology and historical interpretation.* New York: Oxford University Press.

Ryer, C. (2008). NLA-I media statement regarding consensual SM.

Sagarin, B., Lee, E., and Klement, K. (2015). Sadomasochism without Sex? Exploring the Parallels between BDSM and Extreme Rituals. *Journal of Positive Sexuality, 1*(3), 32-36. Retrieved from http://journalofpositivesexuality.org/wp-content/uploads/2015/11/Parallels-Between-BDSM-and-Extreme-Ritual-Sagarin-Lee-Klement.pdf

Saketopoulou, A. (2014). To Suffer Pleasure: The Shattering of the Ego as the Psychic Labor of Perverse Sexuality. *Studies in Gender and Sexuality, 15*(4), 254-268. DOI: 10.1080/15240657.2014.970479

Sandler, J., & Freud, A. (1983). Discussions in the Hampstead Index of the ego and the mechanisms of defense. *Journal of the American Psychoanalytic Association, 31S*, 19-147.

Silverstein, J., L. (1994). Power and sexuality: Influence of early object relations. *Psychoanalytic Psychology, 11*(1), 33-46.

Simon, W. (1996). *Postmodern sexualities.* New York: Routledge.

Sisson, K. (2007). The cultural formation of S/M: History and analysis. In D. Langdridge & M. Barker (Eds.), *Safe, sane and consensual: Contemporary perspectives on sadomasochism* (pp. 10-34). New York: Palgrave Macmillan.

Smirnoff, V. N. (1969). The masochistic contract. *The International Journal of Psychoanalysis, 50*, 665-671.

Southern Baptist Convention. Family statement, March 16, 2010, from http://www.sbc.net/bfm/bfm2000.asp#xviii

Steiner, J. (1982). Perverse relationships between parts of the self: A clinical illustration. *The International Journal of Psychoanalysis, 63*, 241-251.

Stoller, R. (1975). *Perversion: The erotic form of hatred.* New York: Pantheon Books.

Stoller, R. (1991). *Pain and passion.* New York: Plenum Press.

Stoller, R. J. (1985). Chapter 1: Perversion and the desire to harm. *Observing the erotic imagination* (pp. 3-43). New Haven, CT: Yale University Press.

Symington, N. (2002). *A pattern of madness.* London: Karnac.

Tolleson, J. (1996). *The transformative power of stress: The psychological role of gang life in relation to chronic traumatic childhood stress in the lives of urban adolescent males.* Ph.D., Smith College.

Tolleson, J. (2005). *Perversion.* Instructor notes for class lecture. Institute for Clinical Social Work.

Tolpin, M. (1997). The development of sexuality and the self. *The Annual of Psychoanalysis, 25*, 173-187.

Warren, J. (2000). *The loving dominant.* Emeryville, CA: Greenery Press.

Weille, K.-L. H. (2002). The psychodynamics of consensual sado-masochistic and dominant-submissive sexual games. *Studies in Gender and Sexuality, 3*(131-160).

Weinberg, T. (2006). Sadomasochism and the social sciences: A review of the sociological and social psychological literature. In P. J. Kleinplatz & C. Moser (Eds.), *Sadomasochism: Powerful pleasures* (pp. 17-40). Binghamton, NY: Harrington Park Press.

Weinberg, T. S. (1995). Sociological and social psychological issues in the study of sadomasochism. In T. S. Weinberg (Ed.), *S&M: Studies in dominance and submission* (pp. 289-303). Amherst, NY: Prometheus.

Whitebook, J. (1991). Perversion: Destruction and reparation: On the contributions of Janine Chasseguet-Smirgel and Joyce McDougall. *American Imago, 48*, 329-350.

Williams, D., Prior, E. (2015). "Wait, Go Back, I Might Miss Something Important!" Applying Leisure 101 to Simplify and Complicate BDSM. *Journal of Positive Sexuality, 1*(3), 44-49. Retrieved from http://journalofpositivesexuality.org/wp-content/uploads/2015/11/Applying-Leisure-101-to-Simplify-and-Complicate-BDSM-Williams-Prior.pdf

Williams, D. (2015). "Does Social Work Need A Good Spanking? The Refusal to Embrace BDSM Scholarship and Implications for Sexually Diverse Clients. *Journal of Positive Sexuality, 1*(2), 37-41. Retrieved from http://journalofpositivesexuality.org/wp-content/uploads/2014/06/Does-Social-Work-Need-a-Good-Spanking-Williams.pdf

Williams, D., Thomas, J., Prior, E., & Christensen, M.C. (2014). From "SSC" and "RACK" to the "4Cs": Introducing a new Framework for Negotiating BDSM Participation. *Electronic Journal of Human Sexuality, 17.* Retrieved from http://www.ejhs.org/volume17/BDSM.html

Wilson, C. R. (2006). Manners. In C. R. Wilson (Ed.), *The new encyclopedia of southern culture* (Vol. Myth, Manners, & Memory, pp. 96-104). Chapel Hill: The University of North Carolina Press.

Winnicott, D. W. (1969). The use of an object and relating through identifications. *International Journal of Psycho-Analysis, 50,* 711-716.

Winnicott, D. W. (1971). *Playing and reality.* London: Tavistock Publications.

Yin, R. K. (2009). *Case study research: Design and methods, fourth edition.* Los Angeles: Sage Publications, Inc.

Yost, M. (2007). The impact of gender and S/M role on fantasy content. In D. Langdridge & M. Barker (Ed.), *Safe, sane, and consensual: Contemporary perspectives on sadomasochism* (pp. 135-154). New York: Palgrave Macmillan.

www.ingramcontent.com/pod-product-compliance
Lightning Source LLC
Chambersburg PA
CBHW031434270326
41930CB00007B/708